PUSHBUTTON PSYCHIATRY

Updated Paperback Edition

PUSHBUTTON PSYCHIATRY

A Cultural History of Electroshock in America

Updated Paperback Edition

Timothy W. Kneeland

Carol A.B. Warren

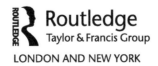

Routledge

Taylor & Francis Group

LONDON AND NEW YORK

Originally published in hardcover by Praeger Publishers, 2002

First published 2002 by Left Coast Press, Inc.

Published 2016 by Routledge
2 Park Square, Milton Park, Abingdon, Oxon OX14 4RN
711 Third Avenue, New York, NY 10017, USA

Routledge is an imprint of the Taylor & Francis Group, an informa business

Library of Congress Cataloguing-in-Publication Data:

Kneeland, Timothy W., 1962–Pushbutton psychiatry : a history of electroshock in America / Timothy W. Kneeland and Carol A.B. Warren.
p. cm.
Includes bibliographical references and index.
ISBN 0–275–96815–4 (alk. paper) hardcover
ISBN 978-1-59874-363-0 (alk.paper) paperback
1. Electroconvulsive therapy—United States—History—20th century. I. Warren, Carol
A. B., 1944– II. Title.
RC485 .K645 2002
616.89'122'0973—dc21 2001036697

ISBN 978-1-59874-363-0 paperback

Contents

Preface

Electroshock (EST), or Electroconvulsive Therapy (ECT), developed during the 1930s in Europe, is an established procedure in contemporary American psychiatry. But it is also extremely controversial, as demonstrated by the diverse (and telling) titles of the many books and articles about ECT since the 1930s—such as *The Miracle of Shock* (Peck, 1974), *Shock Treatment is Not Good for Your Brain* (Friedberg, 1976), *Electroshock: Its Brain-Disabling Effects* (Breggin, 1979), and *Electroshock: Restoring the Mind* (Fink, 1999). This history of electroshock traces both the treatment and its controversies from its origins in ancient electrotherapeutics until the turn of the new millennium.

The story of electroshock in America began thousands of miles and years away from the American continent, in and around the waters of the Mediterranean and the Baltic. Its origins, antedating pushbutton psychiatry by millennia, involved the magical and medical uses of the static electricity in amber and the electrical charge from fish and eels. We follow the thread of the electrical from ancient Greece and Rome to modern America, at times converging with the history of magnetism, with which the history of electricity has frequently been intertwined.

Our task in the chapters that follow is to explore the relationship between electricity and psychiatry from the eighteenth to the late twentieth century in America, against the background of ancient and modern electrotherapeutics. The Western context of electrical medicine is hierarchical and patriarchal, with medical treatment, expertise, and reimbursement the provenance of male physicians and heads of households. In patriarchal medicine, it is mainly men who control others' bodies through the staking of claims to lineage or to esoteric, specially trained, state-licensed, or unique knowledge. It is this grid of patriarchal control upon which the body and mind of the psychiatric patient is interpreted and treated. And the Western medical discourse of the body is itself part of the history of the electrical—and vice versa.

Western medicine began with the writings of the Hippocratics four hundred years BCE. By the time of Galen (ca. 130–200 CE) there were two known forms of electricity available to medical practice: the static electricity in amber and other "electric" stones, and the shock from electric fish and eels. Amber is the general name for a "fossil resin . . . succinite" found—and highly valued—in Europe since prehistoric times (Beck and Shennan, 1991: 16). The Greek name for amber was electron, the electric stone. Thales, around 600 BCE, "found that by rubbing amber it would attract eight substances . . . he reasoned that it had a soul . . . in fact he had only decomposed its natural electricity and established in it an electrical force. Natural electricity pervades all nature, things animate and inanimate. Without its invigorating influence, all life would become extinct" (Ives, 1879: 7).

Amber's enduring associations in the West are with hierarchy, wealth, gender, and healing. Poinar (1992: 1) notes that "Fascination with amber dates back to prehistoric times, when this form of fossilized resin was probably considered to have magical powers and was used for adornment and trade." Archaeological evidence indicates an association with gender as well as class hierarchy: amber daggers have been found in men's graves, and jewelry in women's (Champion, 1984; Beck and Shennan, 1991; Poinar, 1992). Amber (as well as ambergris, a substance exuded from the sperm whale) was used in both amulet and liquid (succinic acid) forms for medical treatment in Greece and Rome (Riddle, 1992a; 1992b), including hysteria in women (Poinar, 1992: 2). The first book written on amber, in 1551, dealt with its medical properties (Poinar, 1992: 3), a focus that continued into the nineteenth century.

Electric fish and eels are found in the Mediterranean and other seas and waters; among the "strongly electric" fish are the electric catfish, the electric eel, and the electric ray. These fish "held the attention of natural philosophers in four epochs—ancient Egypt, classical Greece, Imperial Rome, and post-Renaissance Europe, but passed out of fashion during the Middle Ages and after the Renaissance" (Amberson, 1958: 36–37). Like amber, electric fish have been used in Western medical treatment both nutritionally (Kellaway, 1946: 124) and for their shock. The shock of the electric fish was used by Galen and by Arab physicians for the treatment of a number of ailments, including epilepsy, melancholia, and depression (Wu, 1984; Rudloe and Rudloe, 1993; Schechter, 1983; Neaman, 1976: 13).

From ancient times, philosophers had been fascinated by magnetism (the lodestone) as well as electricity; the property common to both was that of attraction from a distance. Magnetism, like electricity, was used, from prehistoric times onward in Europe, to treat a variety of ailments, including melancholia (Senior, 1983; Krusen, 1942: 22; Thorndike, 1923: 143; Macklis, 1993: 376). And, like electricity, magnetism formed part of the Western language of love, attraction, and sexuality (Macklis, 1993; Murray, 1885: 268). During the Renaissance, natural philosophers designed experiments to explore the properties of amber (and other electric stones) and the lodestone, and the differences between them. In 1600, William Gilbert, in England, published *de Magnete*, a treatise on the properties of amber and other "electrics" and of the lodestone. A half century later, Sir Thomas Browne referred for the first time to "electricity" (Overmeier and Senior, 1992), while in 1660 von Guericke devised the first machine to generate an electrical charge (Rowbottom and Susskind, 1984). It took another hundred years to put generated electricity, in the form of the Leyden jar (see Chapter 1), at the center of medical treatment.

By the time of Columbus and his momentous voyage, electricity and magnetism had been harnessed to the treatment of numerous physical and mental disorders, especially mania, melancholia, and hysteria. The treatment of mental disorder in Western medicine is grounded in the body and its four humors; aimed at the behavioral, rational, emotional, or role-related symptoms of insanity that have troubled family members and puzzled experts throughout recorded history. Ancient electrotherapy for insanity was practiced upon the body, seeking to rebalance its fluids through nutrition; and upon the organs, discharging a galvanic shock through the brain—arguably the site of the soul, emotion, or reason. But electrotherapy was also practiced upon the genitalia, especially in the case of female hysteria. The threads of electricity and the genital treatment of hysteria were not drawn together until the nineteenth century, but the origins of this convergence are found in the Hippocratic and post-Hippocratic gynecologies, and in Galen's widow's treatment.

The Hippocratics and Galen were among the canonical medical authorities whose opinions and practices echoed throughout the Middle Ages and into the modern age of science. From Plato and the Hippocratics came the imagery of women's mental disorder as caused by the wandering womb, a uterus deprived of sexual intercourse and rising in protest into the throat, there to create hysterical symptoms. From the post-Hippocratic gynecologies was derived the practice of clitoridectomy to treat women's mental symptoms (Hanson, 1995), and from Galen its opposite: clitoral or uterine stimulation as a treatment for mental disorder (see Roccatagliata, 1986: 204; Simon, 1978; King, 1993). Used through the middle ages and into the twentieth century, Galen's widow's treatment was one aspect of the control of female sexual response or orgasm in the service of a patriarchal medicine; the outcome of male medical theories rather than female desires (see Chapter 3).

THE STUDY

The intersection of electricity and the body with gender hierarchies is at the center of this history of electrotherapeutics, and forms the background of our interpretation of electroshock in America. Since it is medical experts whose voices have been heard since antiquity, in philosophical treatises and the case history, it is mainly their voices that are heard in this study. And those voices are themselves arrayed within disciplinary hierarchies: ancient philosophers, famous physicians and infamous, published and unpublished experts, specialist gynecologists and andrologists, highly paid private psychiatrists and humble asylum alienists, lay practitioners, quacks, and Royal Society experimental philosophers. The primary sources we use include case histories, medical records, textbooks, and pamphlets—predominantly Anglo-American but also including some French and other European sources. We also use media, novels, ethnographic and interview research, and the Internet for our analysis of twentieth-century EST—the era when patients' voices were at last heard extensively among those of the physicians. In addition to these primary sources, we use secondary works in areas such as the histories of medicine, psychiatry, the body, gender, and anatomy. With Roccatagliata (1986) we use the term "psychiatry"—arguably anachronistic—to denote the medical treatment of disorders of the reason, behavior, or emotions (whatever their presumed etiology).

This is a short history of electroshock, based upon a great deal of primary and secondary data, but highly selective in order to keep the length of the book manageable. We chose examples using two principles. One, we selected the most interesting quotes to epitomize our analytic generalizations; for example, in Chapter 1, John Wesley's excitement about the new electrical experiments. Two, we included rare or exceptional cases to counterpoint or highlight general trends; for example, in Chapter 3, what may be the last twentieth-century appearance of the genitals in the electrical treatment of mental illness (Steinfeld, 1951). We decided not to use footnotes or endnotes; hopefully our readers will be convinced by our narrative and sources of our scholarly credentials.

There are interesting issues of authority, gender, and reflexivity in these sources. As Foucault has noted, the disciplinary "gaze" of patriarchal medicine is leveled at the female (and male) body, framing and classifying it. But at the same time there is another gaze; that of the male physician toward his disciplinary peers, past and present. The case history is shaped not only by the gaze of the physician upon the patient's body, but also by his eye upon the place he would like to occupy within the textual hierarchies of medicine.

In his discussion of Galen, Lloyd (1973) sketches the parameters of Western patriarchal medicine's male-to-male gaze. He notes that "the profession that provided Galen was"—and is—"an extremely competitive one," in which "Galen describes his colleagues as descending to every kind of corrupt practice to build up their own reputations and undermine those of rivals." Galen himself sought to draw boundaries between legitimate physicians and "the soothsayer . . . the mere drug seller . . . and the layman," and tried to persuade his colleagues that the collection of fees for medical care was inappropriate (Lloyd, 1973: 152 and 137). The turn—beginning during the scientific revolution (Jardine, 1999)—from medical claims based on ancient authorities to those based on empirical evidence did not dislodge the commercial and competitive nature of Western medicine and medical publishing.

Thus, well aware of such issues of representation—bedeviling these postmodern times—we make no claim that our history represents, mirror-like, events in the past, nor that it is more than one possible history of EST. We situate our account within the framework of the electrical and the electrotherapeutic rather than the convulsive, while other scholars such as Richard Abrams (1992: 3) and Max Fink (1999) take the opposite approach. Lothar Kalinowsky, the mid-twentieth-century émigré who helped introduce EST to America (see Chapter 3), insisted that "Electroconvulsive therapy . . . bore no resemblance to earlier attempts to use electric current for the treatment of mental illness, such as the Romans' use of electric eels" (1982: 1). Obviously, we disagree.

Our electrical history is arranged part temporally, part thematically, and—since both electrotherapeutics and EST came from Europe to America—it has European as well as American roots. In our Introduction, "Electricity, Psychiatry, and American Culture," we situate the story of EST both in the golden age of the American electrical (the 1870s to the 1900s) and in ancient debates over the nature of the body and its disorders. We focus on the development of the capitalist marketplace during the late nineteenth century as the locale for the development of electrical machinery, the assembly line, and electrotherapeutics. The 1930s invention of pushbutton psychiatry in the EST "buzzbox" was the culmination of European and American fascination with the machine.

Part I, on electricity and electrotherapeutics prior to the era of EST, analyzes the application of electricity to physical and mental symptoms during the eighteenth and nineteenth centuries in Europe (particularly France and England) and America. Chapter 1, set upon the electric stage, illustrates the interplay of science with entertainment during the late seventeenth to late eighteenth centuries, and the association of electrical medicine with gimmickry and quackery. During this era, science gradually superseded entertainment, and the electrical inventions of Americans such as Ben Franklin were linked with the medical electricity of Europeans such as John Wesley in England and Franz Mesmer in France—with innovation and medical applications, like revolutionary politics, going back and forth across the Atlantic.

In Chapter 2, we explore the nineteenth-century American experience with electrotherapeutics for insanity, as the American fascination with electricity came to dominate the landscape of both the real and the imaginary. This was the great age of the insane asylum in America; institutional insanity spread across the nation, gathering hundreds of thousands of patients within its enormous edifices. Both psychiatry and electrotherapy became increasingly specialized during this period, formalizing into numerous organizations and journals. The private electrotherapeutic practitioner treated the upper-middle-class neurasthenic "woman on the couch" (Jordanova, 1989) with local or general electricity, while the asylum alienist threw up his hands in helplessness at the condition of hereditary degenerates, pauper lunatics, and dangerous lower-class men. At the *fin de siècle*, Freud's talking cure changed psychiatric practice, and electrical treatment gradually fell out of favor—until the birth of EST on or around (see Chapter 3) April 15, 1938.

Part II explores the birth, death, and rebirth of electroshock therapy in America in the decades between 1938 and 1999. World War II and the fascist movement formed the context for the Italian birth of EST during the 1930s, which we describe in Chapter 3. The acceptance and use of EST first in Europe and then America was astounding. Initially proposed for "chronic institutionalized incurable" psychotics and schizophrenics, EST during the 1940s–1950s was rapidly accepted in America as a treatment for depressives and neurotics, and equally rapidly displaced alternative convulsive treatments such as fever (see the Introduction). Nevertheless, all was not new: although initial EST experiments often used equal numbers of men and women, it soon became—like its nineteenth-century electrotherapeutic predecessors—a treatment directed predominantly at insanity among women.

Chapter 4 relates the backlash against EST in the 1960s and 1970s, in the contexts of professional rivalries and the patients' rights movement. Patients who had been treated with electroshock against their will fought back, and wrote about it. The voices of patients, first heard in the eighteenth and nineteenth centuries, grew into a chorus during the twentieth: the names of ex-patient writers such as Sylvia Plath and Mark Vonnegut were joined to those of Virginia Woolf and Charlotte Perkins Gilman. Anti-EST psychiatrists— John M. Friedberg, Thomas Szasz, and Peter Breggin—joined textual forces with the ex-patients, as did sociological and media commentators. Subsequent attempts to regulate or ban ECT (as it had by then become known) through the legislative process failed several times during the 1970s and 1980s. But by the mid-1970s, the resurrection of electroshock had begun.

Chapter 5 explores both the resurrection and the 1990s landscape of ECT. Against the background of political and economic movements in medicine—in particular public and private insurance and later managed care—ECT returned as a preferred treatment for a whole range of psychiatric diagnoses. Initially (as in the eighteenth century) a treatment of last resort, the "new and improved" ECT soon became a first resort and even prophylactic treatment during the late 1980s and early 1990s. University hospitals returned to the teaching of ECT, some dusting off old equipment, some investing in new equipment and special wards. The American Psychiatric Association (APA) and National Institute of Mental Health (NIMH) developed new and improved equipment and procedural guidelines; an NIMH conference in 1985 legitimated the "new" ECT technology for the next generation of practitioners. Celebrity ECT patients such as Dick Cavett joined their voices to those of pro-ECT psychiatrists—Max Fink, Richard Abrams—in praise of ECT. And, although the ancient patriarchal hierarchies of electrical medicine were not displaced, something was new: elderly bodies, as well as women's bodies, became the subject of ECT treatment.

The Epilogue closes our story at the opening of the twenty-first century, the third millennium of the body electric, and the second century of pushbutton psychiatry. ECT is in place—for now—as the sole convulsive— electrical psychiatric treatment in America, celebrated or derided on Internet Web sites designed for psychiatric practitioners or ex-patients. But other electric and magnetic treatments, associated with the "new age" of alternative medicine, have appeared upon the fringes—and even into the mainstream—of medical practice: ancient amber has returned in amulet form with its healing powers, and the magnet circles wrists and fingers. We end our story where it began, with the electric body, part of the electric firmament.

BUT DOES IT WORK?

But does it work? Since this, we have learned, is the inevitable question following upon any oral or written presentation of our work, we decided to approach, if not answer it, in this Preface. Since we are not clinicians, but rather a historian and a sociologist, this is not our question. Our question is, rather, what does ECT mean? What does it mean to those who propose, administer, or write about it; from the elderly depressed patient in a university hospital in the year 2001, to the 1980s physician selling $400 tapes of ECT treatments, to John Wesley in thrall to eighteenth-century ethereal fire, to the soul that once animated the bones, adorned with amber jewelry, found in neolithic graves, to the ardent eighteenth-century adventurers seeking the electric eel in South American rivers? These meanings—individual, cultural, and historical—are the burden of our tale.

Acknowledgments

First of all, each of us acknowledges the other; sharing our separate histories of Electroconvulsive Therapy (ECT) made the book, and the experience, all the richer. We brought to the project different aspects of the research and writing process, as well as different perspectives and sources of data; the order of names is, thus, alphabetical rather than representative of senior and junior authorship. We would both like to thank our editors at Greenwood Publishing Group for their interest in the project and the time they took with it.

I thank the librarians and archivists at the Bakken Institute, the National Library of Medicine, and the American Psychiatric Association, who assisted me in putting this work together, and the Pew Foundation and Greenville College, Illinois, for summer funding for work on Chapter 3. I want especially to thank my wife, Laura, who understands all too well how this book became a part of my personal, as well as professional life.

Timothy W. Kneeland

I too want to thank the librarians and archivists at the Bakken Institute for their sponsorship of the early stages of this research, especially Liz Ihrig, and those of the University of Kansas Spencer Rare Books Library in the later stages. Above all, my thanks go to Susan Case of the Anschutz Library, University of Kansas, Lawrence, for her invaluable support of this project throughout the 1990s. Without the help and support of the University of Kansas administrative and secretarial staff, especially Pat Johnston and Penny Fritts of the Sociology Department, and Lynn Porter of the College of Liberal Arts and Sciences, I would not have been able to get this book done—or anything else for that matter. And a big kiss for all my loved ones, especially Ian and Kathi, who make everything possible.

Carol A.B. Warren

Introduction: Electricity, Psychiatry, and American Culture

The story of electrotherapeutics and EST in nineteenth- and twentieth-century America is framed within both the ancient patriarchal culture of the West and the modern age of technology and capitalism. The great transformation in Western material culture was the Industrial Revolution of the nineteenth century, with its final transmogrification of the marketplace into a capitalist form. Electricity was capitalism's source of power, both materially and metaphorically, embodied in the electrical machine. The transformations of the Industrial Revolution were true equally of Europe and America, but were (as all things seem to be) magnified in America. In America the linkage between general cultural themes and medical treatments is particularly clear in the years from Edison's invention of the electrical lighting system in 1879 to World War I, a period in which electricity dominated the public imagination and reinforced patients' acceptance of electrical medicine.

During the last two decades of the nineteenth century, in particular, electricity awed America. With no hint of hyperbole, Henry Adams said that "It is a new century, and what we used to call electricity is its new god" (quoted in Essid, 1993: 10). In the article "Is Electricity Life?" Henry Lake answered, in 1870, that it was; indeed, it was the "very soul of the universe. It permeates all space, surrounds the earth, and is found in every part of it . . . men and women are electrical machines" (quoted in Green, 1986: 197). Electricity—symbolizing natural and supernatural forces, organic and inorganic processes—was a source of awe, and sometimes fear. It was the stuff of magic and Arabian nights (Jackson, 1895: 1–6). It was associated with ideas of social change and progress as varied as the eugenics movement, reform politics, and sexual radicalism (Aspiz, 1987).

One of the most significant arenas of public appreciation for the powers of electricity in the late nineteenth century was the local, national, or international fair. Nearly one hundred million people visited American fairs and expositions between 1876 and 1916. At the fairs, electricity inspired fairgoers with spectacular lighting displays that were often the central attraction (Rydell, 1984: 2). As the motive power of the age, electricity was featured at the World's Columbian Exposition that began with a dramatic lighting of the exhibits on May 1, 1893 (Badger, 1979: 10). Over two and three quarter million people came to see the Columbian Exposition, and *Scientific American* noted that the most visited attraction was the electric building (Essid, 1993: 8).

At these fairs, electricity was presented as an aspect of the machine. Henry Adams conflated electricity with the dynamo and suggested the awe it inspired by commenting that after a time "one began to pray to it" (Adams, 1918: 380). Man (and we use the gender deliberately) has been fascinated by machines since before the Trojan horse revealed its treacherous interior. From the seventeenth-century invention, in England, of the induction machine, electrical machinery has entered into the repertoire of Western scientific medicine. As we will see in Part 1, the invention and use of electrical machinery gained momentum during the eighteenth century in Europe and America, and, by the middle of the nineteenth, had diversified from static to battery-type, galvanic, franklinic, and other types of electricity, machinery, and current. Just as the idea of electricity entranced the American public in the half century after 1870, the idea of the machine was enthusiastically reembraced in the mid-twentieth century, together with the enduring association between electricity, the machine, and the human body.

ELECTROTHERAPEUTICS AND ELECTROTHERAPISTS

From the seventeenth century onward in Europe and America, interest in electricity and the electrical machine was central to the field of medicine as well as popular culture. By the mid-nineteenth century, "electrotherapeutics" was a part of medical terminology in America, and electrical medicine the provenance of specialist, as well as general physicians. Nineteenth-century electrotherapists shared the American fascination with the electrical. One exclaimed, "We are living in an electrical age" (Neiswanger, 1900: 31–32), while another echoed, "The age in which we are living may, with a certain propriety, be called the age of electricity" (Bracket, 1890: 1).

The development of electrotherapeutics in America paralleled the growth of electrical technology and of the capitalist marketplace, and was shaped by medicine's boundary-drawing "professionalization" during that era. In the late nineteenth century, physicians rewrote the history of electrotherapeutics by suggesting that electrical treatments given prior to 1870 were dispensed by quacks and charlatans. Thus Dr. William James Dugan insisted that "Electrotherapeutics has passed from the domain of the charlatan to that of the regular practitioner" (Dugan, 1910: v; see also Frederick Strong, 1908). Physicians such as Dugan organized to preserve their authority over electric medicine and to intervene between patients and treatments, dismissing the "large advertisements of charlatans who advertise electric belts and other contrivances" (Dugan, 1910: 4).

The American marketplace of the late nineteenth century transformed patterns of consumption and production, making medical (including electrical) treatments available, through advertising, for mass consumption. This "democratization" of electrical appliances in the marketplace caused concern among those seeking to create medical specialties in electrotherapeutics, and roused the twin hegemony-maintaining specters of quackery and abuse by laypersons (King, 1892: 43). Some physicians voiced outrage at the "stupidity and ignorance of the public who by electric nostrums, think that electricity is the vital principle itself, and regard it as the great cure-all" (Morton, 1892: 3). Others gave up, admitting that they used electricity only because "patients desire it" (Goelet, 1893: 2). Phelps lamented the power of patient pressure on his practice: "The widespread belief among the laity, that in the latest discoveries in Electro-therapeutics, is found a panacea for all their ills. . . . It had been a potent influence in putting an electrical outfit in many a doctor's office with more or less disastrous results to the cause of Electro-therapeutics" (1894: 224).

A few physicians in Europe and America harked back to ancient amber in their therapies. French physicians Dr. Gerard and Dr. Trousseau in 1842, and Drs. Beaumetz and Abadie in 1879, reported in *Journal des Connaissances Medico-Chirurgicales* on the treatment of female hysteria with various stones and metals, including magnets and amber. Drs. Beaumetz and Abadie applied amber to the temporal lobes of their patients, concluding that metals helped relieve hysterical symptoms, but static electricity was curative (1879: 537). Across the Atlantic there was still some physician interest in the use of amber in medicine, but mainly as an oil or liniment; interestingly, several nineteenth-century handbooks that discussed amber associated it with hysteria and (less overtly) with sexuality. In his *Materia Medica* (1842), John M. Eberle mentioned the use of amber amulets in healing, and proposed the use of oil of amber, which "heats the system and excites the secretions," in cases of hysteria in women and "nocturnal pollution" in men. In treatises later in the century, Buck (1885) and Scudder (1898) dismissed the use of the amber stone in medicine, but recommended the use of oil of amber as a "stimulant" in cases of "nervous affections" such as hysteria (Scudder, 1898: 377 and 642).

By 1898, when Scudder published his handbook, generated electricity was intertwined with the lives and practices not only of physicians and patients, but also politicians and businessmen. There were machines in public places that would, for a penny or nickel, provide a charge of electricity to cure nervous ailments or rheumatism. Congress had a cellar room in the Capitol filled with electrical medical apparatus in the 1880s; the *Electric Review* noted, "The members say it is splendid after they have exhausted their brain power by speechmaking or listening. A great many members take electricity, and some go to the basement every day during the season" (Nye, 1991: 153). Manufacturers took advantage of this public and political fascination with electricity, and generated new machines. Edison cultivated a close association with electrotherapist George Beard for both scientific and commercial reasons. A letter from business manager J.B. Edson to Edison touched upon this theme: "I commend him to you—he could also place many of your instruments among his patients and certificates from him would be of great value—as he is an acknowledged authority on such matters" (Edison, 1991: 321).

While some retailers, including Sears, Roebuck and Co., sold electric belts and other devices through their catalogs to the lay public (see Chapter 2), others advertised to physicians. Jerome Kidder, McIntosh Battery, Pulvermacher, and Waite and Barlett were all successful in having their wares displayed in the medical literature. Other companies sold electrical "self help" books written by physicians but containing pictures and descriptions of their machines. Illustrated catalogs and pamphlets aimed at physicians informed them that they could increase their incomes with electrical machines incorporating marble slabs and elaborate switches and clockwork (Bennett, 1912). Nineteenth-century American electrotherapists were as fascinated by the electrical machines as were their patients (Twiss, 1911: 92). Large static-electrical machines proliferated in medical offices after 1890, leading one physician to hope that "we can locate a machine at every cross-roads in the rural districts and the majority of city offices . . . machines are modernized; the lines are . . . beautiful" (Bartholow, 1890: 169–174). Thus were inscribed the mechanics and electrics of late nineteenth-century American technology onto the human body.

AT THE PUSH OF A BUTTON

With the widespread domestication of electricity during the first third of the twentieth century, electricity lost some of its imaginative powers, while Freudian theory promised a new, psychically based approach to mental disorder. But by the end of World War II there was a renewed interest in electrical machinery in America, based not only on the return of somatic theory in psychiatry, but also on a renewed fascination with the machine, and with the metaphor of "man" as machine. While some émigrés from Nazi Europe brought with them shock machines that reshaped American psychiatric practice, another group of refugees reconfigured the American urban landscape to reflect the machine age.

Linking the rise of pushbutton psychiatry to technologically inspired developments in art, architecture, and literature suggests how deeply the American fascination with machines penetrated American culture. Walter Gropius, Ludwig Mies Van der Rohe, and members of the Bauhaus movement in architecture arrived in the United States during the same time period as Lothar Kalinowsky and other promoters of electroshock therapy (Tallack, 1991: 115). Walter Gropius, moving away from an architectural landscape inspired by the organicism of designers such as Frank Lloyd Wright, sought an architecture adapted to the twentieth-century world of machines (Hughes, 1989: 309). As American psychiatrists pioneered somatic treatments using the electrical machine, advocates of the Bauhaus transformed the spaces where these treatments were given.

The celebration of the machine was an integral component of the enthusiastic adoption of electroshock in America in the 1940s—nicknamed the "buzzbox." Practitioners set to work with these boxes, in Europe and America. One of the originators of EST, Lucio Bini (see Chapter 3) "set to work making big boxes and little boxes with all sorts of curious electrical insides. Until at last he had one about the size of an overnight bag. And this one seemed to do everything he wanted it to do and nothing he didn't" (Ray, 1946: 228). American psychiatrists elaborated new machines and features. In 1945, Douglas Goldman and W.T. Liberson designed a machine that would give a brief shock, while in 1946 Liberson added a feature that regulated the voltage according to the body's "electrical resistance" (Goldman, 1949: 36–45; "Latest News on Shock Treatments," 1947: 30). Other machines focused electricity on one part of the brain (Friedman, 1942: 218–223). The continual introduction of "new features" into the machine, including the switch from metal to wood cases, parallels that of the automotive industry. Interestingly, the machines constructed during the 1940s may have fallen short of the dramatics expected a half century earlier: "Strange as it may seem, we have sometimes been criticized for making our equipment *too simple*. We have been told that it doesn't seem impressive or awe-inspiring; that we need more panel lights, and chrome plating" (*American Journal of Psychiatry*, 1943: iii).

Popular press accounts of EST emphasized the combination of electricity, efficiency, and portability in the machine. The *New York Times* told readers in 1940 that "the electric shock is produced by a small portable electric box" ("Insanity Treated by Electric Shock," 1940: 17). *Science News Letter* accompanied one of its first news articles on EST with a photo captioned "Electroshock Apparatus," showing Kalinowsky and Barrera behind the machine. The text explained, "The complete apparatus is portable and can be carried to a ward and even to a patient's home for treatment," and continued on a utopian note: "It is hoped that the day may come when the man or woman suffering from delusions . . . may some day be simply cured in his own home . . . by a physician who placed two electrodes on the distressed head and then just plugs in an ordinary house current stepped down to the harmless voltage used" (Van De Water, 1940: 43–44).

The EST machine was promoted as preferable to other forms of inducing convulsion precisely because it was electrical, and it was a machine. Machinery, in medicine as in other cultural spheres, was "technically simpler and cleaner" than other, more organic methods (Kalinowsky and Hoch, 1946: 106). And, like most of the household appliances of the times, the electroshock machine operated with the push of a button: "With the dials on the shock machine set to deliver an exact amount of current, the operator simply pushes a button and the treatment is on" (Shyrock, 1947: 61). In many accounts the patient was only so much material to be manipulated by the machine, passively receiving the treatment: "In submitting to the shock, the patient is laid on a bed with his arms and legs fastened and held by four attendants; an adhesive covered tongue depressor is placed between the patient's teeth to prevent biting the tongue. At the push of a button" (Dunham and Weinberg, 1960: 169–170).

Not only had electrical treatment become pushbutton by the middle of the twentieth century, the assembly line had joined the machine as the mode of delivery. During the nineteenth and early twentieth centuries the factory became the major means of production in America, a workplace increasingly streamlined and rationalized. In the age of EST, the metaphor of the machine joined that of the assembly line, and treatments were given to batches of patients in hospitals on particular days and at particular times of the day. One author describes:

> Some twenty men, in bathrobes and pajamas . . . awaiting treatment. . . . Dr. Deutsch, in his long white coat, [stood] at the head of a treatment table surrounded by doctors, nurses, attendants. Behind him on a small table was a metal box about twelve by ten inches. . . . The dripping forceps are clamped over Bevan's head, a pad on each temple. A gag is slipped between his teeth, the five attendants bear down on ankles, knees, hands, and shoulders. Dr. Deutsch reaches out to the box . . . he throws the switch. . . . The eyes roll up, the face pours sweat, throat and chest are inflamed. . . . But when he is rolled out of the room in just sixty seconds flat, the man is blue. . . . Another man walks in—and another—one every few minutes, it goes on all morning. (Ray, 1946: 229)

The EST assembly line still existed during the late twentieth century; Barnes Jewish Hospital in St. Louis was nicknamed "Barnes Jiffy Jolt" by patients because of its assembly line approach to electroshock (Batz, 1996: 21). As in the auto industry, the assembly line had triumphed.

The metaphors of the machine, the assembly line and the marketplace entered the discourses of those who provided electroshock in America at midcentury. Lothar Kalinowsky termed patients "material," and noted that successful treatment enabled them to become "productive" or at least engage in "occupational therapy" (1953: 61). The patient was something to be repaired or engineered, to be restored to productivity. Recalling the fascist context in which EST was invented (see Chapter 3), the psychiatrist became an engineer for a smoothly functioning and trouble-free society. Important social functions were to be restored to the impaired.

THE ELECTRICAL PATIENT: CLASS, RACE, AND GENDER

From its earliest history, electrical treatment has had a variety of associations, through symptoms and diagnosis, with class, race, and gender. During the era of electrotherapy, in the late nineteenth and early twentieth centuries, physicians linked the rise of neurasthenia and hysteria to the development of civilization. The highest classes, the brainworkers, were unable to keep pace with the rate of progress, stressing their brains, which could then be restored by electricity (Beard, 1881: 96–129). The problems of the lower classes stemmed from different sources, such as hereditary degeneracy, and were not amenable to electrical treatment (Tousey, 1921: 519). During the late nineteenth century the "typical American hysteric was a white woman age 16–25" (Hammond, 1871: 630), and the "disease" was common "in white and yellow but never in brown and black" (Dana, 1925: 456). Although some early recipients of EST were brown, black, or lower class, the treatment was most frequently given in private hospitals to middle-class white patients. These patterns continued into the age of EST and ECT, with patients in the 1960s and 1970s generally "middle-class, middle-aged Anglo women" (Babigian and Guttmacher, 1984: 539; Warren, 1987: 23), and after 1980 elderly rather than middle aged (Warren and Levy, 1991).

Throughout the history of electrical treatment gender has been at the center of the hierarchy of electrical patienthood: male physicians electrifying the bodies of women and men, often young, middle-class women and men. During the nineteenth century, the gendered diagnoses most associated with electrotherapy were neurasthenia, at first a male disorder, and then a female one, and hysteria, since ancient times a prototypically female one. Diagnoses that were seen as related to hard work or overwork outside the home were assigned to males, while those that stressed passivity, irrationality, or emotionality were given to females. As one female physician, Mary Putnam Jacobi, put it, "A distinction is often made, based upon the sex and temper of the patient. . . . If this be female, and notably selfish, the case is pronounced hysteria. If a man, or though a woman amiable and unselfish, the case is called neurasthenia" (1888: 63–64). Having neurasthenia was less stigmatizing than the effeminacy of hysteria; people diagnosed as neurasthenic could at least claim class and gender advantages. Alice James, Theodore Roosevelt, Edison's first wife Mary, Jane Addams, and Margaret Cleaves were all diagnosed as neurasthenic at some point during their lives (Haller, 1971: 474; Baldwin, 1995: 116; Rockwell, 1920: 261). After the turn of the century, however (as we shall see in more detail in Chapter 2), neurasthenia became associated, like hysteria, almost entirely with women.

Electrical treatment has been associated from time immemorial, through the uterine concept of hysteria, not only with gender but with sexuality, a theme we introduced in the Preface and develop further in Part I. The application of the electric current in the late nineteenth and early twentieth century was to the body in its entirety, as a nutritional general treatment, and also to specific local sites that included the brain and the genitalia. During this era, as we shall see in Chapter 2, women's reproductive systems were subjected to both electrogalvanic cautery of the clitoris and stimulation of the uterus or external genitalia with electricity or vibration in the name of mental health. Galen's widow's treatment, and the Hippocratic excision of the clitoris, joined with technology to combat female hysteria and other forms of insanity in the electric body.

THE BODY ELECTRIC

Throughout Western history, insanity has been described in the language of behavior, feeling, rationality, and social role, while its origins have been located within the body and/or the disembodied soul or mind. The origins of Western, and thus American insanity—linguistic, theoretical, and practical—are located in patriarchal dualisms and hierarchies. Ancient dichotomies describe insanity: the sane and the insane, the maniac and the melancholic, the curable and the incurable, in the context of the gendered, humoral, and electric body.

Since the days of the Hippocratics, philosophers and physicians have pondered the nature of human anatomy (Laqueur, 1990), and its physical and mental symptoms of disorder—and the electrical has been part of the interpretation and treatment of the body. Greek philosophy proposed a body whose fate was shaped by the universe and its stars, and the four humors that reflected the four seasons and four elements: the dualities of wet and dry, cold and hot, within the fluids of blood, phlegm, black bile, and yellow bile. Although all bodies—women and men, slave and free, young and old—were composed of the same four humors, the different place of bodies in the great chain of being, and in the cosmos, was reflected in different humoral configurations and quantities (Hippocrates, 1931: 281).

The quantity, quality, and balance of these humors, together with the configuration of stars at birth, and the "airs, waters, places" of the environment, were responsible for wellness and illness as well as temperament. And the humors—together with the brain—could turn personality and behavior into excess, and thence madness. While a sanguine, happy temperament was promoted by blood, and laziness by phlegm, black bile was responsible for a melancholic temperament. Defects in, or excessive amounts of one of the humors, its isolation from the others, or abnormal excretion, could turn the melancholic temperament into melancholia. People whose brains were "maddened through bile are noisy, evil-doers, and restless, always doing something inopportune. These are the causes of continued madness" (Hippocrates, 1923: 177). Medical definitions of insanity were in ancient Greece, as they are today, intertwined with the proprieties of behavior in a given culture. What constituted insanity in the Hippocratic corpus, 25 centuries ago, is familiar to us today: "visual and auditive hallucinations . . . wild talking . . . folly . . . excessive calmness . . . excitement . . . sadness, fear . . . tension at the precordium . . . strange behavior . . . nightmares during sleep . . . attacks of suffocation . . . unfounded worries . . . not recognizing familiar things and feeling confused" (Roccatagliata, 1986: 166). The classifications of insanity used in ancient times have come down to us (multiplied and subclassified) into the present: the ravings of mania, the sadness of melancholia, the fits of epilepsy (today classified as a physical disorder), the hereditary helplessness of idiocy, and the mysterious afflictions attendant upon hysteria, the wandering womb.

During the late nineteenth and early twentieth centuries, the metaphor of the human body as a kind of machine was popular among the lay public and electrotherapists. Practitioners of electrotherapy such as Steele (1871), Hutchinson (1875), Britten (1875), and Dugan (1910) proposed that "man" was but an electrical machine and disease a disturbance or diminution of the electrical forces in the system. Thomas Edison wrote that the human body was a machine that needed a life force, analogous to electricity, to run it (1948: 5). For W. Boyce, the nerves of the body mimicked electricity in the wires of a house, or those of the telegraph line (1880: 68). The cessation of the electrical current caused a breakdown of the machine, while the interruption of the electricity in the human body caused physical or mental disease.

In nineteenth-century medical theory, the mechanism by which the human machine became mentally disordered was through the operation of the nervous system. Chemist George Frederick Barker suggested that the nerve force and electricity were the same (1880: 112–118). For Morrill, electricity penetrated molecules, maintained life, and rejuvenated the "vital force" (1871: 110–112), while Smee published a work on the "voltaic mechanism of man" (Rowbottom and Susskind, 1984: 69). From these mechanical and electrical premises, scientists and physicians traced the cause of nervous disease to electrical breakdown (Clark and Jacyna, 1987: 159).

Treatments practiced upon the body reflect current theories of the "nature" of that body (or soul): talk therapy for disorders of the mind; aromas to tempt the wandering womb back into place; changes in the "airs, waters, places" of the environment; nutrition or pharmaceuticals to alter the fluids; purging to eliminate toxins or excess humors; exorcism to drive out demons; water to cool or heat the overheated or overchilled anatomy; surgery to remove brain or genital lesions responsible for mental symptoms. Electricity healed the electric body, functioning to discharge excess electricity or restore its deficiency, a model echoed in magnetic treatment.

The diagnoses most closely associated with electrical treatment in ancient and medieval medicine included epilepsy as well as hysteria, melancholia, and mania. Epilepsy has been intertwined with both insanity and electricity in the West throughout the centuries, its symptoms seen, prior to the 1900s, as similar to the "fits" of the hysteric (Temkin, 1971). The Hippocratics "pointed out a sort of balance between epilepsy and melancholy; if there was epilepsy, there was no melancholy, and vice versa . . . mania is cured if convulsions arise" (Roccatagliata, 1986: 164–165). This "incompatibility" theory reappeared in the twentieth century in the work of Meduna (see Part II).

Over the centuries, in Europe and America, many theories of the place of electricity in the human body, and of the medical application of electricity to the human body, have appeared and disappeared. Some of these theories and applications can be traced from ancient times to the late twentieth century, such as the local application of electricity (from amber, fish, or machinery) to the brain. Others we note in passing, and perhaps note their passing. Among the uses of electricity that have come and gone before and during the era of electricity in America are the nutritional, electric sleep, and electric light.

The Hippocratics recommended the ingestion of the flesh of the electric fish as one treatment for symptoms of physical and mental disorder. This idea was reborn in the heyday of nineteenth-century American electrical treatment for mental and physical disorders, since one theory of the action of electrical treatment upon the body was nutritional. Beard and Rockwell (1881), the "Deans" of American electrotherapeutics at the *fin de siècle* (see Chapter 2), claimed that electricity had a "tonic" effect by gradually improving nutrition (Beard and Rockwell, 1881: 218). Like the humoral physicians of old, a number of nineteenth-century physicians were obsessed with eliminatory functions; symptoms for mental disorders such as neurasthenia and cerebral hyperaemia included dyspepsia, constipation, or incontinence.

The belief that electricity "vitalized" the body so that it could assimilate and eliminate properly was not confined to Beard and Rockwell. The idea is echoed in the work of chemist George F. Barker, inventor Thomas Edison, and S. Weir Mitchell of "rest cure" fame—and by practitioners deemed to be outside professional boundaries, the so-called "quacks" who sold electrical and magnetic salves and liniments. Although the origin of mental disorder might be nervous, afflicted individuals became worse as their metabolism broke down under the influence of overwork, underwork, or overindulgence. These patients needed to be restored by the nutritional influence of electricity upon the cells. Practitioners of nutritional electricity aimed the current at the torso, along the spine or stomach rather than the brain. Indeed, some nineteenth-century electrotherapists believed that electrifying the brain was dangerous and perhaps deadly (Britten, 1875: 30).

Electronarcosis or electric sleep, associated with Arsene d'Arsonval's and Stephan Leduc's experiments with electroanaesthesia in France in the 1890s and 1900s, is the opposite of the jarring, violent electric shock to the brain (Senior, 1984; Tousey, 1921). In electric sleep, the patient diagnosed with depression or schizophrenia receives continuous electricity to maintain a state of unconsciousness, returning to consciousness after the application of the current is discontinued (Senior, 1984; Tousey, 1921). There were European and American trials of electrosleep as an alternative to EST in the 1940s. In 1948 Harvey J. Tomkins of the Veterans Administration wrote to the medical director of the American Psychiatric Association (APA) saying, "Electronarcosis is being used increasingly in our hospitals judging from the number of requests for machines, we have heard of no untoward results" (Tomkins to Blain, October 15, 1948, Blain Papers). Although electrosleep was widely used only in the USSR (Senior, 1984), Rowbottom and Susskind (1984: 195) indicate that during the 1980s in America there was an "increase in the literature . . . [and] considerable interest in electronarcosis" at the same time that ECT was returning to dominance in the arena of electrical psychiatry (see Chapter 5).

Electric light treatment enjoyed a brief heyday of interest in the era of the electrical in Europe and America (Taylor, 1983: 281). In England, asylum superintendent F. Pritchard-Davies experimented with "polychromatic electric light" in the treatment of insanity, using blue light to control "nervous excitement" and red light for "nervous depression." He claimed that "violent maniacs" were calmed by the "blue room," but that the "red room" was unsuccessful (Pritchard-Davies, 1877: 344). He concluded that the success of his "photochromatic treatment" was attributable to "moral influence," one of the theories proposed in the 1950s to explain the effects of EST. Pritchard-Davies' comments on electric light treatment echo a cyclical model of medical invention—invention, submergence, and reinvention—that also describes the history of electrotherapeutics: "I do not intend making any attempt to give the history of this line of treatment. I am satisfied that it is very old, and has doubtless been tried, forgotten, and reintroduced, as often as have most other things thought to be new" (1877: 344).

The body electric traversed the spaces between the Hippocratic corpus and the age of electricity in America, linking the ancient hierarchies of class (or status, or citizenship), race, age, and gender to physical and mental symptoms and treatments. The relationship between electricity, psychiatry, and American culture is in part an ancient one, with European roots, and in part one of the New World, shaped by a set of peculiarly American materialisms and metaphors. In the tale that follows, we explore the continuities of hierarchy and patriarchy, and the changes in technology, political economy, and physician training and organization, in the electrical treatment of mental disorder in America—and the eventual triumph of electroshock. To rephrase an old saying, "*Plus ça change, plus c'est la meme chose; plus c'est la meme chose, plus ça change.*"

PART I

THE ELECTROTHERAPEUTIC ORIGINS OF PUSHBUTTON PSYCHIATRY

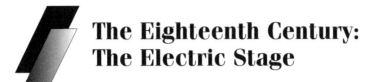

Chapter 1

The Eighteenth Century: The Electric Stage

[F]or deep hysterical cases . . . the patients [should] be simply electrified, sitting on cakes of rosin, at least half an hour morning and evening, then begin to take small sparks from them, and afterwards give them shocks, more or less strong, as their cases require, always beginning with gentle shocks. This method seems very rational.
—John Wesley (Ferguson, 1775)

The eighteenth century in America, as in France and Britain, was a time of profound political and social change, with electrotherapeutics, as well as politics, in ferment on both sides of the Atlantic. Although the individual most closely associated with the electrical in this century was the American Benjamin Franklin, many of the other contributors to the century's electrical innovations were European. The intensity and rapidity of communication between America, Britain, France and other countries made electrotherapeutics (and magnetism) a trans-Atlantic enterprise. This chapter, then, interweaves the American with the European, especially the Anglo-French electrical experience.

In the early part of the century, electrical inventions and discoveries built upon the writings of Gilbert and his successors. In 1709, Frances Hawkesbee made an incandescent bulb. Charles Dufay in 1733 proposed the existence of two types of electricity, "resinous" and "vitreous," while Stephen Grey tested and wrote papers on conduction and insulation during the 1720s (Hankins, 1985: 54–55). In his work, Grey joined eighteenth-century electrical experimentation to the human body, as the practitioners of healing with amber and fish had done in premodern times. In 1730, Grey "electrified a boy of eight or nine . . . probably the first human being to be electrified intentionally. The boy was suspended face downward in a horizontal position by hairlines that hung like swings from hooks driven into the beam of Grey's room. The excited [glass] tube was held near the boy's feet, and a leaf of brass was attracted by the boy's face to a height of 8–9 inches" (Rowbottom and Susskind, 1984: 4).

The invention of the Leyden jar at midcentury, and the work of Luigi Galvani and Alexander Volta at the end of the century, set the stage for the expansion of the electrical during the nineteenth. The Leyden jar permitted the storage of electricity and the generation of stronger shocks than older machines. John Wesley attributed the invention of the Leyden jar to Mr. de Muschenbroek, professor of natural philosophy at Leyden, in 1746 (Wesley, 1790: 13), while Rowbottom and Susskind refer to the "nearly simultaneous discovery" of "the first electrical condenser" to Muschenbroek in 1746 and von Kleist at the end of 1745 (1984: 7–10).

The eighteenth century saw a renewed interest in electric fish and eels, especially following the invention of the Leyden jar. In Europe, Francisco Kedi and his pupil dissected torpedos, concluding that the electric organ of this fish was a type of muscle (Wu, 1984: 600). An "electrical circle" was formed which included Joseph Priestley, Ben Franklin, and John Walsh (Wu, 1984; Benjamin, 1989). Studies of the European torpedo concluded that the opposite sides of the fish represented opposite electrical poles, suggesting positive and negative electricity to Ben Franklin (Wu, 1984: 601). At the end of the century, the electrical discoveries by Luigi Galvani, a medical professor at Padua, and Alexander Volta, a professor of natural philosophy at Padua, advanced the technology of the electrical beyond the Leyden jar. In his experiments with the electrification of frogs, Galvani claimed to have proved the presence of a "nervo-electric fluid" as the basis of animal life. In his correspondence with Galvani, Volta "at first accepted Galvani's doctrine of animal electricity as a stupendous discovery" (Rowbottom and Susskind, 984: 43), but later developed a different theory of electricity and became Galvani's rival. Volta himself became known as the inventor of the first battery prototype, a giant metallic coil.

These discoveries and experiments reverberated across the Atlantic to America, and back. The most important eighteenth-century American figure in the history of electricity is Ben Franklin, whose electrical experiments were published in 1751 in the *Gentleman's Magazine*, and widely disseminated in England and France as well as America. Franklin suggested that electricity and lightning were the same phenomena, and he devised an experiment to prove this: the famous kite experiment. He also developed a theory of electricity suggesting that certain bodies had an excess or positive amount of electricity and were therefore positively charged, while others had a deficiency of electricity or were negatively charged (Cohen, 1990: 66–109). Like many electrical inventors in the eighteenth century, Franklin practiced electrical medicine, treating both men and women for a variety of ailments (Franklin, 1961: 503; 1962: 525; 1968: 27–28).

These discoveries and experiments demonstrated, for the eighteenth-century natural philosopher, the "link between power, knowledge, and electricity" (Aspiz, 1987: 30–31), and harnessed the power of the electrical to a degree unprecedented in prior centuries. By the early nineteenth century, electricity had become associated with mastery over the human body, and a sexualized, masculine dominance over nature. In 1802, Davy commented that science in general, and electricity in particular, had "bestowed upon man powers which may almost be called creative, which have enabled him to modify and change the beings surrounding him, and by his experiments to interrogate nature with power, not simply as a scholar, passive and seeking only to understand her operation, but rather as a master active with his own instruments" (quoted in Aspiz, 1987: 31). The use of sexual metaphors to describe electricity and science, as well as their objects of study, became commonplace between the late eighteenth and late nineteenth centuries (Benjamin, 1989).

There was a darker side to electricity in the eighteenth century: its conflation of human and machine, and life and death. In stories such as that of Frankenstein, technology appears as the key both to man's (used advisedly) control and loss of control over life and death (Joerges, 1990). In the preface to *Frankenstein*, published in 1817, Mary Shelley described the genesis of her concept in eighteenth-century electrical experimentation: "Perhaps a corpse would be reanimated; galvanism had given token of such things: perhaps the component parts of a creature might be manufactured, brought together, and endued with vital warmth" (1951: xxxiv). And it was not only in the imagination that women and men of the eighteenth century attempted animation and reanimation. Giovanni Aldini, nephew of Luigi Galvani, was among those who—like Mary Shelley's protagonist—attempted to revive the dead (typically, the corpses of executed criminals) by electrical stimulation. These goings-on were the subject of satire in the eighteenth and nineteenth centuries, by a public made uneasy as well as hopeful and amazed by the new science:

> For he ('tis told in public papers)
> Can make dead people cut droll capers,
> And shuffling off death's iron trammels,
> To kick and hop like dancing camels.
>   (see Kuhfeld, 1991: 3)

If the completely dead could not be revived by electricity, perhaps the near-dead could. In the late eighteenth century Wilkinson (1792) quoted a description of a 20-year-old woman patient evocative of Ophelia, the symbol of women and madness (see Showalter, 1985):

"She exhibited," says he, "a figure of death-like sleep, beyond the power of art to imitate, or the imagination to conceive. Her forehead was serene, her features perfectly composed. The paleness of her color, her breathing at a distance being also scarce perceptible, operated in rendering the similitude to marble more exact and striking. The position of her fingers, hands and arms was altered with difficulty; but they preserved every form of flexure they acquired." (p. 55)

Wilkinson added that after electrical treatment, the woman was reborn "into a perfect state of health," adding that the case "seems to be worthy of being recorded, both on account of the uncommon symptoms that attended it, and the relief obtained by electricity" (1792: 60).

THE ELECTRICAL PHYSICIAN

Historians trace the use of electricity in eighteenth-century medicine to Professor Johann Gottlieb Krueger, chair of medicine at the University of Halle, who was asked by a student in 1740 what might be the uses in medicine of the new science of electricity. Krueger suggested that it might be most useful in the treatment of paralysis, a theme that continued throughout the century (Licht, 1967: 3). In 1747, Jallabert, a Swiss experimental philosopher, used electricity to stimulate muscles, while Lovett, a clerk at Worcestershire Cathedral, used electricity to treat hysteria (Rowbottom and Susskind, 1984: 16–19). Electrical medicine was practiced in American by physicians and scientists, including Ben Franklin (Cohen, 1990: 37).

A range of instruments and methods were used, in Europe and America, to electrify patients' bodies. In England, Lovett electrified patients insulated on cakes of resin, administered "light shocks" to, and drew sparks from, patients (Rowbottom and Susskind, 1984: 19). In France, Maudyt immersed patients in electrical fluids in baths (Sutton, 1981: 584). Other methods of application included the electric breeze, electric feather, electric friction, and the use of the Leyden jar with water (Licht, 1967; Rowbottom and Susskind, 1984). The most "heroic" method, called "commotion," caused muscular contractions and could result in blindness or death (Licht, 1967: 14), while some of the other treatments caused pain.

Throughout the century, electrotherapists sought to improve their machinery and techniques in order to minimize the dangers posed by electricity. Lowndes contrasted the late eighteenth- with early eighteenth-century uses of electricity in medicine, in a manner reminiscent of contrasts made by practitioners between 1940s and 1990s ECT: "That prepossession in favor of Electricity as a certain remedy for every disease incident to the human body, which prevailed a few years ago, seems to have generally subsided. . . . The modern practice of Electricity rejects those violent modes, such as strong shocks etc., which accompanied its first introduction into medicine. All the good effects that it is capable of producing are now found to result from more gentle applications" (Lowndes, 1787: 9–13).

In comparison with other treatments available in the eighteenth century, Lowndes saw electricity as less dangerous and with less problematic side effects, a position also taken by late twentieth-century psychiatrists in relation to ECT treatment of the elderly (see Chapter 5): "Electricity is entirely free from . . . pernicious effects. It can be applied to any particular diseased part, independent of the rest of the body, and when diffused through the system in general, it permanently enlivens the spirits, and increases the vital function, without ever being succeeded by dejection" (Lowndes, 1787: 12).

Eighteenth-century electrotherapists sought to understand the physical and curative properties of the electrical. Some, like John Wesley, saw electricity as a life-force associated with the universe and with the divine. Others thought that perhaps its effect was psychosomatic. Haygarth concluded from his placebo study (see below) that the power of electrical devices was mental rather than physical: "Such is the wonderful force of the imagination!" (1800: np). Ben Franklin, who was ambivalent about electric medicine, proposed that either walking to his house for the treatment, or the hope aroused by the procedure, accounted for its success (Taylor, 1983: 281). Still others, including Aldini (1803), thought that trauma to the brain or other parts of the body was responsible for the mental cures effected by electricity. Whytt referred to the curative effect of blows, noises, and whips on epileptics, and cited the case of "a girl who was cured of epileptic fits arising from melancholy, by firing a gun at her bedside, just as she was coming out of one of the paroxysms" (1787: 677).

On both sides of the Atlantic, the eighteenth century was an era not only of scientific experimentation, but also of the formal organization of the knowledge so gained. The locus of scientific work in Europe had shifted during the seventeenth century from the church to the universities and royal societies; the first four scientific societies were formed between 1657 and 1700 (Freedman, 1975; Heilbron, 1979; Jardine, 1999). During the eighteenth century, both the work of these societies and the proliferation of journals in Europe and America encouraged the rapid development and dissemination of knowledge related to electricity and electrotherapeutics. Between 1750 and 1789, 26 papers dealing with medical electricity appeared in one of these journals alone, the French *Journal de Medecin* (Kellaway, 1946: 134).

This formalization of scientific and medical knowledge led to boundary disputes in electrotherapeutics as in many other specialties. Scientists, theologians, and physicians seized upon the electrical and the magnetic, but so did others deemed to be (by contemporary or later commentators) empirics, or even quacks. As John Wesley noted, the wonders of the new electrical experimentation were such that asserting the "truths" of the science of electricity itself might be grounds for the charge of quackery: "Of the facts we are absolutely assured: although they are of so surprizing a nature, that a man could not have asserted them a few years ago, without giving up his reputation" (Wesley, 1759: A2). What Wesley said of electricity in general in the 1750s, could also be said of electrotherapeutics: this all sounds far too good to be true. The claims of quacks such as Giovanni Pivati of Venice, who proposed that electricity could be bottled as a sort of drug, did not help the reputation of mid-eighteenth-century electrotherapists. The Abbe Nollet traveled from France to Italy to investigate Pivati's claims, finding them to be invalid although perhaps not deliberately fraudulent (Rowbottom and Susskind, 1984: 18). Despite the aura of potential quackery, physicians, electricians, and others continued to experiment with medical electricity throughout the century.

Electrical physicians staked their claim to legitimacy on the grounds of diagnostic expertise, which could be acquired only through medical education. Cavallo (1780: 6) characterized nonmedical electrotherapists as "ignorant persons." William Rowley, who toured through France, Germany, and Italy in the 1790s visiting hospitals that used electrical treatment and criticized nonmedical electricians for their lack of diagnostic training, wrote:

As many writers on electricians have not been physicians, some allowance should be made for their want of accuracy and precision in nominating and treating many diseases, of the nature of which they have sometimes been mistaken, and, of course, introduced doubtful information; indeed, so doubtful, that men, deeply versed in the science of medicine, have scarce credited many relations published; with all these imputations, however, they have done much service to society. (1793: 444)

One American electrician seemed to know his place. He wrote that "for my own part, being but a young electrician I can have very little to say with respect to the medical part [of electrical treatment]. But, as far as I have had experience, I shall here relate the facts" (Ferguson, 1775: 120).

Other boundary disputes revolved around the distinction between legitimate scientific and medical practices on the one hand, and quackery on the other. These disputes centered on two issues: the legitimation of the practitioner by emerging formal organizations (university training, royal society membership, journal publication), and his (or, sometimes, her) apparent moral character. Even if formally qualified, a practitioner could find himself ostracized by colleagues as a quack if he seemed to engage in shady practices; practices which included advertising, collecting enormous fees, claiming universal success, and the sexualization of treatments (Porter, 1989; Porter and Hall, 1996). Among eighteenth-century electrical and magnetic practitioners eventually deemed quacks by their peers were James Graham in England, Franz Mesmer in France, and Elisha Perkins in America.

James Graham operated a "Temple of Health" in London, featuring a large, electrified bed intended to stimulate fertility in those couples who paid to disport in it (Rowbottom and Susskind, 1984). Invoking the ancient belief in the necessity of the female orgasm for conception, he advertised his "Celestial or Magnetico-electric bed . . . the first and only ever in the world" in dramatic language:

Any gentleman and lay desirous of progeny, and wishing to spend an evening in the Celestial apartment, which coiton may, on compliment of a [fifty pound] banknote, be permitted to partake of the heavenly joys it affords by causing immediate conception, accompanied by soft music. Superior ecstasy which the parties enjoy in the Celestial Bed is really astonishing and never before thought of in this world: the barren must certainly become fruitful when they are powerfully agitated in the delights of love. (quoted in Porter and Hall, 1996: 110)

Franz Anton Mesmer (referred to in some eighteenth-century texts as "Friedrich" or "Anthony") also epitomized the link between sexuality, gender, and the magnetic in his mesmeric treatment. Mesmer's theory of "animal magnetism" formed the basis of his treatments, which involved magnetic tubs filled with iron filings, swooning young women, and strong men prodding them with magnetic wands (Mackay, 1841; Sutton, 1981). Mesmer thought that the magnetic was "almost the same thing" as the electrical (Mackay, 1841: 322), and proposed that ill health was the result of the interruption of magnetic fluid through the body, an interruption that could be halted by his and his assistants' interventions.

Mesmer's reception by his clientele on the one hand, and by established medicine on the other, is illustrative both of the eighteenth-century formalization of science, and of the important linkages between the two sides of the Atlantic. In 1778 in Paris, his cures of women hysterics—which sometimes involved comas and convulsions—seemed miraculous. By 1783 "both electrical medicine and mesmerism had large, important and adoring clienteles" (Sutton, 1981: 392) and perhaps competing ones. Following his surge of popularity, Mesmer was labeled a quack, in part because of an investigative committee that included Ben Franklin. By the time of his death in 1815 his treatments had been defined as "imaginary" by the French Academy of Science, on grounds that included excessive fees and the "licentiousness" of his treatments. Sutton (1981) notes that the success of Maudyt and his electrical treatment, and the failure of Mesmer and his magnetism, can be traced to their different fates at the hands of legitimating authority. Yet, despite the discrediting of Mesmer, mesmerism continued to have some adherents in Europe and America into the nineteenth century and beyond (see Darnton, 1968).

One of the most notorious American quacks of his time, Elisha Perkins, was known for his development and direct sale of "Metallic Tractors," which had nothing in common with the farm machinery that comes to mind today. Perkins' tractors consisted of two small metal rods, one of brass and one of iron, which were to be rubbed on the body of those afflicted with disorders to draw off a "noxious" excess of electricity. The appeal of the rods was not, like Graham's bed or Mesmer's salons, erotic; it seems to have rested upon their small size, ease of purchase (although costly) and application, and connection with ancient yet powerful theories of electrical and magnetic polarities. Even George Washington bought a pair (Greenway, 1989: 51). Perkins' tractors were so popular (by his estimate he sold 3,000), that a "cult," "perkinism," was given his name—and Perkins was expelled by the Medical Society of the state of Connecticut as a quack (Schechter, 1983: 35).

However, this was not the end of the tractors. Perkins' son Benjamin took the tractors to England and Denmark (150 cases of them), publishing *Experiments with the Metallic Tractors* (Perkins, 1799). Benjamin noted that the tractors, together with "Directions for their use in families . . . may be had of the Editor, at his house in Leicester Square, price five guineas the set" (Perkins, 1977: xvii). Dr. Charles Cunningham Langley of Bath also sold the tractors, and published "A view of the Perkinean electricity" in 1798 and 1799. In response to Langley's report, Dr. John Haygarth devised a controlled experiment of sorts, in which some patients with swellings were treated with real tractors, and some with wooden ones made to look like the originals. Equal numbers of those in the control and experimental groups (all but one in each) reported improvement in their symptoms (Haygarth, 1800; Hunter and Macalpine, 1963).

THE ELECTRIC STAGE

Although showmanship and dramatics were part of the reason for the labeling of Graham, Mesmer, and Perkins as quacks, showmanship and dramatics were an integral part of eighteenth- as well as seventeenth-century science and medicine (Jardine, 1999). Following upon Grey's experiments, the electrification of the human body became a source of public entertainment as well as edification—a development that eventuated, by the end of the century, in boundary disputes between "real science" and dramatic spectacle. Schechter describes the "parlor games" of the eighteenth-century electric stage:

Electricity was recruited for social amusement. To the great mirth of onlookers, participants vied with each other to produce such configurations as "halos," "electrical kisses," "electrical rain," and so on. Of these parlor games the *pièce de resistance*, which simultaneously illustrated the conductivity of the human body, was to suspend a youngster on hair cords from the ceiling and elicit some harmless sparks from the body. When the child's heels were touched with a charged tube, bits of copper leaf were attracted to the head. (1983: 22)

In arenas larger than parlors, these electrified human dramas were even more astonishing. In France:

Reports of experiments . . . read to the Royal Society in 1746, included accounts of passing the shock through an incredibly large number of persons joining hands, with an operator holding the phial at one end of the "curve" and another touching the wire at the opposite end. On one occasion in a demonstration before the king organized by the Abbe Nollet, 180 guards were said to have been made to jump simultaneously; on another, an entire community of Carthusian monks at Paris, linked together by iron wires, were reported to have made the distance traveled by the shock over 5,000 feet (1.5 km.). (Rowbottom and Susskind, 1984: 809)

Medical electricity was part of this electric stage. In the United States from the 1740s onward, electrical experiments were presented for public edification. Boston hosted a series of yearly electrical entertainments lasting about two months (Morse, 1934: 365). On August 18, 1749:

The Gentleman who has been entertaining us with a Course of very curious electrical Experiments, has also applied the Electrical fire to the human frame with remarkable and speedy Success, in curing the Tooth-Ach, Pain in the Head, Deafness, Pains in all the Limbs, which had been so violent as to take away the use of them, Pain in the Stomach, Swellings of the Spleen, Sprains, Relaxation of the Nerves, etc. The most remarkable are the two following instances, viz: One Samuel Milner, who for three Years past could not lift his Head without putting his Shoulder out of joint, by a few Applications of the Electrical fire has met with a perfect cure. A Negro Boy, about sixteen Years of Age, who has always been so Deaf as scarcely to hear the loudest Sounds, has by the same Means been brought to hear, when spoken to in a common Tone of Voice. (Morse, 1934: 366)

Accounts of the electrical stage are implicitly gendered, with the entertainer, natural philosopher, cleric or physician in charge a male, and the subject or patient a child, a man (perhaps a "Negro Boy" as in one of the Boston cases), and sometimes a woman. References to the electrification of women on the electric stage seem at times sexualized as well as gendered, despite Cavallo's caveat concerning electrical vibratory treatment: "To these mild, and even pleasing operations, the most timid or nervous of either sex need not fear to submit" (1780: 19–20). On the list of twenty electrical wonders displayed by Ebenezer Kinnersley in Boston in 1751 was "The Salute repulsed by Ladies Fire; or Fire darting from a Lady's Lips, so she may defy any person to salute her" (Morse, 1934: 369). During the Abbe Nollet's journey through Italy "to rout out quacks and fakers," Veratti electrified a young woman for Nollet and his companion, a cardinal. She did not perform as advertised. Veratti's explanation of the failure must have piqued their curiosity: " 'Monsignors,' he said to the cardinal, 'it is because we could not electrify her in your presence as she should be electrified' " (quoted in Heilbron, 1979: 354). Or perhaps it was because of the class-inferior bodies of Veratti's experimental subjects, "a valet and two servingwomen," that proper electrification failed. After his experience with Veratti, Nollet concluded that neither "Children, Servants, or people of the lower Class" could be admitted to his experiments (Schaffer, 1992: 347).

Several themes in eighteenth-century electrical medicine are exemplified by the experiences of John Wesley, the Protestant divine, in England: the transatlantic connections (in this case with Ben Franklin), the combination of technology with transcendence, and the designation of electricity as (close to) the universal cure, the desideratum or panacea. Like many of his contemporaries, Wesley was introduced to electricity by witnessing staged experiments. In November 1747 he wrote in his diary of his introduction to the glass globe: "I went with 2 friends to see what are called the Electrical experiments . . . who can comprehend, how fire lives in water, and passes through it more freely than through air? How flame issues out of my finger, real flame, such as sets fire to spirits of wine? How these, and many more as strange phenomena, arise from the turning round a glass globe?" (Wesley, 1958: 73). Wesley's diaries document his increasing fascination with electricity. In February 1753, he referred to reading Dr. Franklin's letters on the nature of electricity. A few days later he recorded his own trials of electrical medicine. That month he treated four patients with electricity, one a paralytic, and three with abdominal or stomach pain. By November 1756, Wesley had purchased an electrical "apparatus" from Ben Franklin, and had opened a clinic (eventually he had three) for the provision of electrical treatment to the poor of London (Wesley, 1958).

As a cleric, Wesley was interested in the relationship of electricity to the divine. Like many eighteenth-century thinkers (and their predecessors), he came close to identifying electricity with the life force, and with God and the universe. In an oft-quoted passage, he referred to electricity as:

the general instrument of all the Motion in the Universe. . . . For in Truth there is but one Kind of Fire in nature, which exists in all Places and in all Bodies. And this is subtle and active enough, not only to be, under the great Cause, the secondary Cause of Motion, but to produce and sustain Life thro'out all Nature, as well in Animals as in Vegetables. . . . This great machine of the World requires some such constant, active, and powerful Principle, constituted by its Creator, to keep the heavenly Bodies in their several Courses, and at the same Time give Support, Life, and Increase to the various Inhabitants of the Earth. (Wesley, 1790: A3)

This quote is from a 1790 edition of Wesley's work on electrical medicine, *Desideratum, or Electricity Made Plain and Useful by a Lover of Mankind, and of Common Sense*. In this treatise, Wesley described nearly 100 cases (about half men and boys, half women and girls) of electrical treatments of mental and physical ailments, all of which were recorded as successful. The "desideratum" to which the title referred was that universally desired treatment for illness that had been sought by philosophers throughout the centuries. He wrote that "there cannot be in nature any such thing as an absolute *panacea*: a medicine that will cure every disease incident to the human body. If there could, Electricity would bid fairer for it, than any other thing in the world . . . still one may upon the whole pronounce it the *desideratum*, the general and rarely failing remedy, in nervous Cases of every kind (palsies excepted); as well as in many others" (1790: v–vi). Wesley concluded that "perhaps there is no nervous distemper whatsoever, which would not yield to a steady use of this remedy" (1790: 43). Secular practitioners of electrotherapy were inclined to agree, sowing the seeds of what was to become, by the twentieth century, a full-fledged electrical psychiatry.

ELECTRICAL PSYCHIATRY

Throughout the century, the use of electricity to treat human ailments included those disorders—insanity, mania, melancholia, and hysteria—whose symptoms included the emotional and cognitive. Kreuger's legendary Halle lecture was attended by Gottlieb Kratzenstein, who tried electricity on himself and found that it allowed him to sleep better. He proposed the use of electrotherapy with those suffering from mental as well as physical illness: "Electrotherapy would do good, not only in physical but mental patients whose wealth, worries and anxieties prevent them from sleeping at night. Since the blood is made thinner and less viscous through rapid circulation, electrification must be an excellent remedy in thickened blood and hypochondriasis, and in women with hysterical conditions" (quoted in Licht, 1967: 6–7).

Practitioners on both sides of the Atlantic experimented with the electrical treatment of madness, many claiming dramatic success. Some, such as Wesley and Lovett, saw electricity as a kind of panacea, while others (like some twentieth-century ECT physicians) proposed it as a last resort. In England, Symes described sending his servant as an "Out Patient to the Infirmary with 'Hysteric Fits' "; after several months without improvement "I proposed electricity to her" (1771: 58–59). He alternated electrical treatment (passing shocks through her heart, and back and forth over her right and left shoulders) with cold baths, and indicated that "at the writing this, December 24 1764, she continues in perfect health" (p. 60).

The ancient disorder of hysteria remained predominantly an affliction of the female gender and its humors during the eighteenth century, despite emergent theories of nerve afflictions (rather than the uterus alone) as a source of symptoms. Whytt, in England, proposed that hysterical and hypochondriacal disorders were caused by nerves "irritated by acrid humors" with "a fault either in their coats, their medullay substance, or the brain and spinal marrow, from which they all proceed" (1765: 104–105). Like a number of European and American practitioners in the eighteenth century, he treated hysterical females with electricity; if caused by "obstructed menses," he claimed, hysteria could be treated by "electrifying them, and drawing the sparks chiefly from their thighs" (Whytt, 1765: 395). Francis Lowndes (1787), a self-described "medical electrician of St. Paul's Church Yard in London," treated women for amenorrhea using an "enormous electrical machine" (Rowbottom and Susskind, 1984: 27–28).

In America, Cadwallader-Evans (1754) described a case of a 14-year-old girl who suffered from "an obstruction of the menses," cramps, convulsive fits, and "a whole train of hysteric symptoms for some ten years" (pp. 83–84). By 1752 she had decided to try electricity, since nothing else had worked, and went to Ben Franklin for treatment. In a letter to Cadwallader-Evans she described the treatment and its results, which, since the voices of patients were mostly unheard prior to the nineteenth century, is worth quoting in full:

At length my spirits were quite broke and subdued with so many years affliction, and indeed I was almost grown desperate, being left without hope or relief. About this time there was great talk of the wonderful power of electricity; and as a person reduced to the last extremity, is glad to catch at any thing; I happened to think it might be useful to me. . . . I received four shocks morning and evening; they were what they call 200 strokes of the wheel, which fills an eight gallon bottle, and indeed they were very severe. On receiving the first shock, I received the fit very strong, but the second effectually carried it off; and thus it was every time I went through the operation; yet the symptoms gradually decreased, till at length they intirely [*sic*] left me. I staid [*sic*] in town two weeks, and when I went home, B. Franklin was so good as to supply me with a globe and bottle, to electrify myself every day for three months. The fits were soon carried off, but the cramp continued somewhat longer, though it was scarcely troublesome, and very seldom returned. I now enjoy such a state of health as I would have given all the world for, this time two years. (pp. 84–86)

That these patients were women is not unusual; case studies of the use of electricity for hysteria by Lovett (1756), Wilkinson (1792), and others were also of women. At times, electricity was also used to treat men suffering from hypochondria, a disease seen as the equivalent of female hysteria, with its organic origins in the spleen or "alimentary canal" (Whytt, 1765: 104–105). The patient deemed mentally disordered was so deemed in part through a refusal or inability to perform properly within eighteenth- (and later nineteenth- and twentieth-) century structures of gender, family and sexual roles. Male patients were those who could not, or would not work (if they needed to), or who moped and sulked womanishly in their homes instead of functioning in the public world where they belonged—or, perhaps, they raved dangerously around the community, threatening life and limb. Women patients had gone sexually or domestically awry, who were sexual when they should be unresponsive (occasionally vice versa), or who did not perform their proper wifely, motherly, or daughterly duties. These were vulnerable or hysterical women, and dangerous or idle men.

MADWOMEN: VULNERABILITY, DOMESTICITY, AND HYSTERIA

During the eighteenth (and nineteenth) century in Europe and America, vulnerability to mental derangement was associated with civilization, education, the urban, and the female gender (and perhaps genitalia) counterposed to the sturdy sanity of the rural, uneducated male peasant. In France, Beauchêne commented that "Men . . . are also tormented by nervous maladies, but less than women, among whom the ravages are deadly. . . . It is demonstrated by the comparison of rural women with those from the town, that most often the 'vapours' have their origins in temperaments enfeebled by lively passions, by an active imagination, and by too many lively pleasures" (1783: 248). Women who were not only upper class and urban, but who also ventured to educate their minds, were particularly vulnerable, since their mental exertions threatened the functioning of their reproductive systems, a theme taken up with a vengeance during the next century (Shorter, 1994: 66–69).

The sites of electrical treatment for hysteria during the eighteenth century were often the legs, arms, shoulders, and spine; Wilkerson, for example, "passed several of the strongest shocks he could well collect" from the "Leyden phial" he used on a hysterical woman's legs, arms and spine (1792: 59). But by the turn of the eighteenth century there were signs of the electrical renaissance of Galen's widow's treatment, although referencing menstrual obstruction rather than sexual frustration as the cause of symptoms and target of intervention.

In 1803 Carpue, a London "Surgeon," wrote of the use of electrical shock to the "pubis" and "In the region of the uterus" (pp. 56–57). In 1802, a French author described, in Latin (the preferred language for delicate subjects), the "shameful practice" of "tickling a woman to stop her hysterical fits" (Shorter, 1992: 92). In 1800, John Birch published an essay on the use of electricity in the treatment of female genital "obstructions," assuring the reader that there was no "indelicacy" to the "mode of treatment" (p. vii). He described the electrical treatment, which used a Leyden jar and two glass rods he called "Directors." These rods were placed

below the peak of her stays . . . the wheel is turned and the shock passes through that part of the Pelvis which is included between the directors. . . . The nerves and vessels [of] the uterus must be affected by the passage of the electrical fluid. (pp. ix–xi)

Apparently Birch knew, and disapproved of, the sexual implications of genital treatment. He noted that "when obstruction is . . . attended with symptoms which require relief, the application of *shocks* are [*sic*] often very improper" (p. xiii), adding defensively, "I hope that no imputation of harboring a secret can be imputed to me; for that is a crime" (p. xv).

Domestic roles were the crucial issue for many late eighteenth- and early nineteenth-century women patients, and electricity was often the treatment of choice. In America, Thomas Brown reported in 1817 on the electrical treatment of his family of troubled women: "My Wife had, for several years, been afflicted with pain in her side, and was also subject to cramp, also hysteric fits. One of my daughters had long been subject to returns of nervous headache, and another was very weak and debilitated, apparently inclined to a consumption, And as long as is this list, we have all been restored to health, by the use of Electricity" (n.p.). A few years earlier, American physician T. Gale (Rowbottom and Susskind, 1984: 29) reported a case history reminiscent of the "mad housewife" gender troubles of ECT patients in the twentieth century (Warren, 1987), troubles which included not taking care of household or child, revulsion from the husband, and anorexia. A young woman, brought to Gale by her mother, was "terrified at the sight of her husband, with whom she had lived in perfect cordiality, until she became insane . . . she was emaciated almost to a skeleton, deep dejection of spirits, gloomy and melancholy" (Gale, 1802: 126). Gale subjected the woman to electrification:

I used all the address in my power to ingratiate myself into the number of her friends, which consisted then of her mother only. . . . Her husband came to the house—I observed her terror—I laid hold of this opportunity to gain upon her feelings; I would not suffer him to come nigh her, pretendedly so; it had the intended effect. To be brief, it was not long before I was able to persuade her to take a little wine; after this, under the appearance of entertainment we got her to the machine. (Gale, 1802: 127)

Electric treatment restored her to her proper place within the family: "All that gloominess of mind was dispelled and she gradually assumed the appearance of cheerfulness; her digestion was promoted, and she began to take nutricious [*sic*] food freely. To be short, in four or five weeks she was able to unite with her husband again in keeping house" (Gale, 1802: 127).

MADMEN: DESPAIR, DANGER, AND IDLENESS

Male electrical patients were of several dispositions; the hypochondriacal man whose symptoms were similar to those of the female hysteric (Whytt, 1765), the violent and dangerous madman afflicted by mania, or the sad, melancholic male reduced to idleness and unable to support his family. Like vulnerable or undomestic women, troublesome male patients were referred by their families to electrical physicians. Gale was not so kindly to the dangerous or violent male patients who caused trouble for their families as he was toward his women patients. He described the treatment of two "madmen" with electric shock. Mr. Olcox, a "tinman" who had cut his own throat, was referred to Gale by his family. Gale "forced him to the machine like a bullock to the slaughter. . . . I observed his habit was firm and sanguine, his pulse very turbulent; I administered exceedingly heavy shocks upon him" (1802: 128). The other man was also brought by his family:

A young man . . . came to me, and informed me that his father was crazy. . . . His family had become much alarmed, and was on the eve of chaining him . . . he told them that the devil said he must kill a daughter of his . . . [the family] brought him forward sometimes in a waggon, and sometimes out of it; several people assisted, but they could not keep his clothing upon him, for he was mad indeed. By the time he was brought to the machine, which was a very costly one, I expected he would break it to pieces; but there being about twenty men to assist, we got the chains to him, and as I did not expect we should all be able to get the second shock upon him, I charged the machine as high as I thought he could bear, and live through. . . . I would have mentioned his name, but it slipped my memory. (Gale, 1802: 129–130)

Gale claimed at least temporary improvement in both these cases.

While Gale in America electrified dangerous and raving madmen, John Birch, surgeon to St. Thomas's hospital in England, treated withdrawn and melancholic males. He electrified four men with melancholia: a warehouse porter "in a state of melancholy, induced by the death of one of his children" who became worse after the treatment; a public singer contemplating suicide; a man of 26 with a "moping melancholy"; and a "laboring man" who had attempted to hang himself (Birch, 1799: 550). After the first series of electrical shocks passed through his head, the public singer talked to Birch about "a wish he had to impress me with the change which the first operation made in his life" (1799: 550). The "porter of the India warehouses" was not working when his wife first referred him to Birch:

He had been two months afflicted. . . . He was quiet, would suffer his wife to lead him about the house, but he ever spoke to her, he sighed frequently and was inattentive to every thing that passed; his appetite and sleep were moderate, his body regular, and his pulse weak and slow. I covered his head with a flannel and rubbed the electric sparks all over his cranium; he seemed to find it disagreeable but said nothing. On the second visit, finding no inconvenience had ensued, I passed six small shocks through the brain in different directions. As soon as he got into an adjoining room and saw his wife, he spoke to her, and in the evening was cheerful, expressing himself as if he thought he should go to work again; I repeated the shocks in like manner on the third and fourth day; after which he went to work. . . . In the latter end of August, 1791, the woman again applied to me; her husband had continued well until that time, but then had a recurrence of his melancholy without any proximate cause. As he had apparent feverish symptoms, I did not think him in a fit state for the electric shock; I therefore advised him to apply for medical aid, and to the hospital, if he grew worse, as I was leaving town. I am unacquainted with the sequel. (Birch, 1799: 548–549)

As Birch's parting advice to the public singer indicates, during the nineteenth century treatment for mental illness was dispensed by practitioners in their own homes and clinics but also in hospitals and asylums.

ELECTROTHERAPEUTICS IN THE ASYLUM

Some electrical medicine was practiced in private physician and electrician practices during the late eighteenth and early nineteenth century, and some (especially in Britain) in institutions such as clinics for the poor, hospitals, and asylums. John Wesley provided electrical treatment to the poor in his London clinics; perhaps to continue his work, the London Electrical Dispensary was opened in 1793, treating about 300 patients a year. Middlesex Hospital, St. Bartholomew's Hospital, and St. Thomas's Hospital—where John Birch was surgeon—acquired electrical machines during the 1760s and 1770s (Rowbottom and Susskind, 1984: 23–28).

These institutions adopted the modern scientific practice of keeping records of patients, treatments, and cures. In Britain, the London Electrical Dispensary reported that about half its yearly cases were cured, and others benefited (Rowbottom and Susskind, 1984: 28). In France, l'Abbe Bertholon (1786) reported on electrical treatments and cures listed by the physicians of the Faculté de Paris. His figures for mental disorders are: for epilepsy, 89 treated and 42 cured; for "nervous affections," 22 treated and 10 cured; for hysteria, 9 treated and 4 cured; for "madness," 7 treated and 3 cured. Bertholon also reported that two women who became pregnant during the course of the treatment gave birth to very strong and healthy offspring, foreshadowing nineteenth-century themes in electrical sexual eugenics (see Chapter 3).

Galvani's nephew Giovanni Aldini experimented with electrical psychiatry in the insane asylum. He persuaded asylum superintendents in several parts of France to allow him to try the effects of galvanism on otherwise "hopeless" lunatics afflicted by "melancholy madness" (Aldini, 1803: 113). Of the two men for whom Aldini claimed a cure, one was Louis Lanzarini, a 27-year-old farmer confined in a lunatic asylum at Boulogne (1803: 114). This case is interesting both because of its detailed description of the treatment, and because of its parallels with Cerletti and Bini's "first" (see Chapter 3) EST treatment in 1938:

I at first administered the Galvanism gradually, forming the arc by means of the hands. Lanzarini, in a state of the utmost dejection, viewed the apparatus and the company present with his eyes fixed and motionless. When interrogated by the physicians and myself in regard to the origin of his malady, he gave laconic and confused answers, which seemed to indicate a great degree of stupidity and derangement. I first moistened his hands and formed an arc with the pile at different heights, to accustom him to endure the action of the apparatus. No change, however, was produced in the patient by this operation. I then repeated the experiment, placing his hands, moistened with salt water, at the bottom of the pile; and conveying an arc from the summit of the pile to different parts of his face, moistened with the same solution. A change was soon observed in the patient's countenance, and his whole demeanor seemed to indicate that the degree of his melancholy was somewhat lessened. (Aldini, 1803: 115)

There are other parallels with Cerletti and Bini, including the electrification of the brain, the reaction of the attendants to the treatment, and the restoration of role as a primary aspect of the "success" of the treatment (see Chapter 3). After several more days of experimentation on Aldini's part, and apparent improvement of Lazarini, Aldini decided "to administer the Galvanism even to the substance of the brain" (1803: 116–117). This part of the treatment was less successful; Aldini commented that "the novelty of the remedy is sufficient to excite a clamor against it, and awaken the prejudice of the assistants, who will even wish to proscribe it before it had been tried" (1803: 120). But treatments did continue, and eventually Lanzarini was returned to his proper (lower-class male) place in society:

On his leaving the hospital, I carried him to my house, that he might be fitted by proper nourishment for resuming his former occupations. He remained with me eight days in the quality of a domestic, during which time he was exceedingly tractable, and performed his duty with great care and attention. (Aldini, 1803: 118)

Many of the concerns surrounding ECT in America can be found in these accounts of electrical medicine in the eighteenth century, including Aldini's: these accounts, in turn, echo the humoral and pneumatic theories of ancient Greece and Rome. Electricity's apparent triumph over paralysis and death did not survive the nineteenth century—it had been found to be no cure for the deanimation of the human body. But it continued in its triumph over gendered deviance, used by male physicians in America, as in Europe, to constrain the behavior of dangerous or useless men, and of women who sought to be useful outside their restricted roles as wives and mothers. Electricity formed one part of the psychiatric straitjacket within which hysterical women and melancholic men were confined both by their families and within the expanding insane asylums of nineteenth-century America.

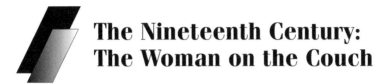

Chapter 2

The Nineteenth Century:
The Woman on the Couch

If the application is made in the office, the patient removes the tighter articles of clothing and lies on a couch; if at home or in a hospital, he or she is entirely undressed and laid in a blanket. A gentle current must always be used at first in a new case, especially in nervous or apprehensive individuals, its strength being gradually increased until satisfactory contractions are produced with a minimum of pain.

—G. Betton Massey, 1889

Between the first and last decades of the nineteenth century, electricity moved from the arena of the religious and universal, subtle fire and ether, to that of the secular and technological. Although still marvelous, as evidenced by its reception at the world's fairs, electricity was, by the 1890s, also harnessed to the pedestrian and domestic worlds of street lighting and household labor (Nye, 1991). Electrotherapy followed suit, the humoral innovations of the early eighteenth century giving way to a clinical, systematized set of practices. After the end of the Civil War, although scholarly communication about electricity continued to cross the Atlantic, electrotherapeutics became independently established in the United States.

Electrical innovation and experimentation in the nineteenth century flourished in the hands of male electricians, scholars, and physicians, who extended, during the first part of the century, the work of Galvani and Volta. In 1831, Michael Faraday combined the electrical and the magnetic into the electromagnetic coil, by which direct current was transferred into alternating or faradic current (Taylor, 1983: 281; Harman, 1982: 31). After alternating current was introduced, electricity could be transmitted for long distances, and was rapidly centralized throughout the nation. This centralization not only laid the foundation for electrified households, but also enabled the direct-sale of electrical appliances for medical purposes in the late nineteenth and early twentieth centuries (Nye, 1991; Overmeier and Senior, 1992).

By the end of the century, there were several types of electricity and electrical device available to the medical practitioner. Static (or "frictional" or "franklinic") electricity, while overshadowed by more sophisticated technology, was used occasionally, alongside galvanism and faradism (Beveridge and Renvoize, 1988: 159). Shock treatment using the Leyden jar was less frequently used than during the eighteenth century (Rockwell, 1891: 161). These electricities were applied generally or locally, through the skin, by electrodes placed on the head, in a sinusoidal bath, by the hand, by a brush, or in bathwater—to name only a very few of the alternatives available (Beveridge and Renvoize, 1988: 159).

During the nineteenth century, electrotherapeutic experimentation resonated with various emergent scientific theories and practices. At midcentury, "Having found that complicated electrical charges take place in a human frame, we may necessarily expect that electricity should be an important remedial agent" (Smee, 1849: 83). Electrical treatment was proposed as rational, scientific, and particularly adapted to the body's "newly discovered" chemistry and neurology. In 1874, Jewell and Bannister wrote that electrotherapeutics "in the hands of a regular physician" promised "a truly rational and scientific treatment of morbid processes and conditions. . . . Certainly no other [treatment] seems to offer more from the alliance of physical and physiological laws, or is more suggestive in view of the important questions of psycho-physics and biology, which are occupying the attention of the scientific world at the present time" (pp. 210–211).

"Scientific and rational" theories of the effects of electricity on the organism remained, however, as varied as they had been in the eighteenth century (and would be with twentieth-century ECT), from the cell-nutritive effect of general faradization (Beard and Rockwell, 1881), to later theories of the power of suggestion or moral effect of the treatment (Valenstein, 1986: 25; Lewis, 1900: 321). Beard even implicated the harnessing of electricity itself as a cause of mental illness: he saw Thomas Edison's inventions as stressing the "change, speed and complexity" of the nervous system and precipitating neurasthenia (Armstrong, 1991: 307).

Early nineteenth-century electrotherapeutics had much in common with eighteenth-century experimentation: accounts are occasional and unsystematic. Together with Gale (1803) and Birch (1803), discussed in the last chapter, Brown (1817), Everett (1817), and Carpue (1803) recounted various trials of and successes with electrical treatment of many physical and mental disorders, including hysteria, epilepsy, and melancholia. Shadrack Ricketson, "Physician in New York," referred to electricity, in 1806, as a "powerful stimulant" that was "frequently used of late, both as a preventive and a cure of many diseases" including epilepsy and suppressed menses (p. 190).

European and American use of electrotherapy accelerated in the 1850s, especially in France and Germany. Guillaume Duchenne, who in 1855 published *De l'electrisation localisée*, stimulated muscle fiber with faradization, detecting—and photographing—nerve-muscle damage and hysterical paralysis (Rowbottom and Susskind, 1984: 71, 103). The systematization of electrotherapeutics in America began at about the same time, with the publication of William F. Channing's *Notes on the Medical Application of Electricity* (1849). In 1858, Alfred C. Garratt published *Medical Electricity*, "the first full-scale textbook of electromedicine" according to Roth (1977: 237). Charles Morgan translated the works of the European electrotherapists and brought them to the United States during the 1860s (Rowbottom and Susskind, 1984: 104–105). By the 1870s in America, Gumplowicz and Klotzberg (1874), among others, were reporting favorable results from many hundreds (rather than just a handful) of cases of the electrical treatment of hysteria and other insanities. By 1880 all kinds of physicians were exposed to the possibilities of electrotherapeutics, from asylum keepers to private practitioners.

ELECTROTHERAPY AND ASYLUM ALIENISTS

As in previous centuries, private practice was one site for the electrical treatment of insanity; the hospital or institution another. But during the nineteenth century, lunatic asylums grew and spread across the American landscape, dominating small towns and villages with their imposing Gothic structures. At the beginning of the century, asylum alienists hoped for a cure for those within asylum walls, perhaps through the "moral treatment" pioneered in France. But by the end of the century, Darwinism in England, and theories of "hereditary degeneracy" in France (Dowboggin, 1991), had rendered the intractable "pauper lunatic" the main inhabitant of the American asylum—with electricity wasted upon his unsuitable class or ethnic body.

The expansion of the European and American asylum during the nineteenth century was accompanied by a search for new theories and treatments of mental illness, and electricity was among the approaches used. Dr. Golding Bird established an Electrotherapeutic Room at Guy's Hospital in 1836 where he used a Leyden jar and a galvanic electric battery; chorea and hysterical paralysis were among the ailments treated (Bird, 1860; Althuis, 1860: 200; Morus, 1992). American asylums were more guarded about electrical treatment than their English counterparts; while employed "sporadically" by American alienists including Francis Besant Bishop (1899), Alfred Tennyson Livingston (1899), and Irwin Neff, electricity was not used routinely by asylum keepers (Neff, 1896–1897: 322–324). Leading neurologist Silas Weir Michell confronted asylum attendants for their neglect of electricity in an address to the fiftieth annual meeting of the Medico-Psychological Association in 1894 (Mitchell, 1894).

Nevertheless, asylums did experiment with electrotherapy in America as well as in Europe. Beard and Rockwell described the use of electricity at New York State's Women's Hospital (1881: 424) and at the Alabama Asylum for the Insane, whose superintendent Dr. Bryce said that it was useful in "hysterical insanity, in primary dementia, and neurasthenia" (Beard and Rockwell, 1881: 438). "Electricity in the form of sparks, shocks and fluid . . .

and shocks through the cranium" was used at New York Hospital in the early nineteenth century (Russell, 1945: 18).

The nineteenth century was a period of specialization and formal organization in medicine, both in and out of the asylum. In 1844, asylum alienists organized as the Association of Medical Superintendents of American Institutions for the Insane (AMSAII), with the *American Journal of Insanity* as their official organ (APA, 1944; McGovern, 1985: 1–2). The creation of organizations and journals by the alienists facilitated the publication of articles concerning the causes and treatment of insanity—and thus, in time-honored fashion, the status of the alienists themselves (Grob, 1994).

The theories of insanity proposed by these men were various, including psychological, phrenological, and other somatic etiologies. Samuel Woodward, head of the Worcester State Asylum from the 1830s to the 1850s, developed a cognitive theory based on wrong mental associations that then had to be "corrected." The lifestyles of the poor were implicated in their disorders, especially excesses such as intemperance, masturbation, overwork, faulty education, extreme religious enthusiasm, jealousy, and pride (Grob, 1994: 58). Control, regulation, and discipline (a variation of moral treatment) were the keys to the treatment of the inmates of the pre-Civil War asylum (Galt, 1870: 80–103). Astonishing cure rates were proposed for this treatment: Samuel Woodward claimed 82–91 percent, while Dr. Todd at the Hartford Retreat claimed 90 percent (Grob, 1962: 420; Bockoven, 1956: 167–194).

By the 1870s, however, notions of curability were fading. Pliny Earle, one of the thirteen founders of the ASMAII, attacked the superintendents' "cult of curability" by claiming that they inflated their cure rate by counting in temporary recoveries (1876–1877: 483). It was not until the asylum came to be made up mainly of permanent residents that the cure rates fell; by 1870, the Utica State Asylum reported a doubled population and a falling recovery rate (*American Journal of Insanity*, 1870: 338; McGovern, 1985: 152). Seventy-seven new state asylums were constructed between 1860 and 1890, with officials increasingly using facilities for persons suffering from long-term chronic illness such as dementia. New York state opened the Willard Asylum exclusively for chronically insane paupers (Dwyer, 1987: 2).

Treatments in American asylums by the 1870s consisted of pharmacology, labor, and perhaps entertainment, reflecting prevailing beliefs that the causes of mental illness were somatic and probably intractable. Brain lesions, heredity, and other aspects of the bodies of the poor and immigrants were proposed as the source of insanity. In an unpublished paper presented at an 1870 ASMAII conference, Isaac Ray of the Utica asylum claimed that the Irish were less curable than other ethnic groups because of their "low order of intellect," and "imperfectly developed brains" (Annual Meeting, October 1870: 157). Only the aging Thomas Kirkbride expressed astonishment at Ray's contentions.

As in the twentieth century, nineteenth-century mental patients could be admitted voluntarily to mental hospitals, or committed against their will. Involuntary commitment came under attack during the 1860s and 1870s in the face of published work critical of asylum practices. A series of exposés of patient abuse at the Bloomington Asylum appeared in the *New York Tribune* between 1869 and 1876 (Bell, 1980: 46). Persons concerned with the issue of wrongful commitment (of the upper classes) to asylums wrote books on both sides of the Atlantic, including Englishman Charles Reade's 1863 novel *Hard Cash*, and Elizabeth Packard's *The Prisoners' Hidden Life, or Insane Asylums Unveiled* (1870). Mrs. Packard was committed after a quarrel with her husband over theology, and her case became a national scandal (Bell, 1980: 46; Tomes, 1984: 291). As a result of these and other publications, commitment practices were altered in Illinois, Rhode Island, and Massachusetts, and the U.S. Congress held hearings on the issue—a process to be repeated a century later, as we shall see in Part II.

NEUROLOGY, QUACKERY, AND ELECTROTHERAPY

The new specialty of neurology, developed in Europe and brought to the United States in the 1860s, revived the hope of psychiatric practitioners both for a cure of insanity and for an improvement in their own public standing. Neurology, carved from the German rationalist and French empiricist traditions, also symbolized American technological and scientific expertise (Blustein, 1981: 242). Neurology dealt with organic disorders such as paralysis, locomotor ataxia, and chorea; such syndromes filled William Hammond's *A Treatise on Diseases of the Nervous System* (1871). Neurologists also saw "nervous" and insane cases on an outpatient basis, believing that both were physical diseases treatable somatically. They used therapeutics such as diet, tonics, rest, and electricity to treat the milder forms of mental illness (Blustein, 1979: 174). And war, as it so often does, stimulated psychiatric innovation. Hammond, surgeon general of the Union Army during the Civil War, set aside separate wards in the Turner's Lane Hospital of Philadelphia for diseases and injuries of the nervous system (Adams, 1952: 171).

Battle lines were drawn between asylum alienists and neurologists after the Civil War over the care and treatment of the insane. Neurologists such as George Beard, William Hammond, S. Weir Mitchell, and Edward Spitzka attacked asylum attendants as unscientific and ignorant, and claimed the right to investigate asylum practices. Hammond was well known for his involvement in a series of court cases aimed at asylum keepers, his call for a supervisory board to oversee asylums in New York state, and his role as a defense legal expert—pitted against prosecution alienists—in courtroom insanity cases (Blustein, 1981: 250–262). For their part, the alienists charged that men such as Beard were incompetent judges of insanity (Everts, 1880: 229–237).

A number of neurological societies were founded in the decades after the Civil War: the New York Neurological Society in 1870, the New York Society for Neurology and Electrology in 1874, and the American Neurological Association in 1875, which adopted the *Journal of Nervous and Mental Disease* as its official publication. By the third half of the nineteenth century neurology had triumphed over the alienists in the quest for scientific respectability, and with the triumph of neurology came the electrical.

Despite the success of neurology and electricity, however, the issue of quackery in electrical medicine had not disappeared. The electrical treatment of insanity in nineteenth-century America took place within the confines of a continuing debate concerning the legitimacy of electrotherapeutics. As in the eighteenth century, the inscription of boundaries between electricians and physicians, empiricists and theoreticians, entertainers and healers (Morus, 1993), and legitimate and quack practitioners continued. The midcentury distinction between electricians and physicians is illustrated by a pamphlet (1846) and book (1849) jointly authored by a Boston doctor, William Channing, and a self-described "magnetical instrument maker" or "electrician," Daniel Davis. They described the use of electricity in cases of "madness," especially "hysteric epilepsy, connected with derangement of the uterine functions," and proposed (Davis adding modest disclaimers as a nonphysician) that electricity was a "vital stimulant" (1849: 131).

Although many neurologists such as James Jackson Putnam, Samuel Webber, Charles Kastner Mills, and William Herdman first obtained positions at hospitals or taught in colleges under the title of "electrician," this term was still used throughout the nineteenth century to denote nonphysician and perhaps questionable practitioners. Even by the 1870s, some physicians complained that the requisites for legitimacy—formal training in diagnosis, and theoretical (rather than simply empirical) knowledge—were often lacking among electrotherapists. Jewell and Bannister wrote in 1874 that "Still, the practice of electrotherapeutics is yet largely empirical; and the amount of professional ignorance on the subject, even among otherwise well-informed practitioners, is something astonishing" (pp. 209–210).

"The practice of electro-therapeutics" was associated not only with neurologists and electrotherapists, but with other European and American theories of anatomy and insanity. Among these was phrenology, based on the early nineteenth-century brain researches of the Germans Franz Joseph Gall and Johann Spurzheim. Phrenology enjoyed considerable popularity during the mid-nineteenth century among American asylum superintendents, but soon came to be dismissed as pseudo-science, if not outright quackery (Scull, MacKenzie, and Hervey, 1996: 98–99). Phrenologists located the causes of mental symptoms in the body, using both humorally-based diagnoses and "faulty cerebral organization" in their model. While some phrenologists favored bloodletting or leeches (Coombe, 1834: 282–283) or moral treatment

(Spurzheim, 1833: 238) for the cure of insanity, some proposed electricity (see, for example, Uwins, 1833). American phrenologists also wrote of the electrical nature of sexuality and reproduction, representing sexuality as an electromagnetic emanation or fluid that gained strength if not expended (Aspiz, 1987: 145–152; Porter and Hall, 1996). Like Galen and his predecessors and successors, these phrenologists—among a host of other American eugenicists and sexual reformers—proposed that infrequent, mutually orgasmic episodes of marital coitus were the only route (given hereditarily nondegenerate parents) to healthy offspring (Porter and Hall, 1996).

But phrenology was not the only theory linked with quackery. Throughout the nineteenth century, the charge of quackery was leveled by some electrotherapists at others. Jewell and Bannister, for example, insisted that electrotherapeutics must be "in the hands of a regular physician" (1874: 208). They criticized, as an exemplar of the irregular type of physician in whose hands electricity should not be, Dr. Arthuis of Paris, who:

> pays very little attention to scientific principles . . . his method consists, rather, in a kind of homeopathic medication by various substances which, he assumes, he is able to introduce through the "pores of the skin" by means of the electric current; his ideas being a modification of those of Beckinsteiner, more fanciful, even, than the original. (Jewell and Bannister, 1874: 214)

Electrical medicine itself was considered quackery by some nonelectrical physicians. Those labeled quacks in print sometimes fought back in print—in their very own journals. In an article coyly entitled "Quackery Must be Put Down" in the *Eclectic Medical Journal*, John Skelton M.D., MRCS, "Consulting Physician to the Northampton Botanic Dispensary" satirized the anti-quackery forces (1858), while in the American "phreno-mesmeric journal" *The Zoist* the contributors ironicized their treatment at the hands of mainstream medicine (1848, see also below).

On the boundary between legitimate medicine and quackery are practices which twentieth-century historians and social scientists refer to as "folk" or "alternative" medicine, reflecting the liminality of such practices as homeopathy, osteopathy, chiropractic—and at times electrotherapy. With liminality comes gender difference—mainstream and quack medicine generally associated with male practitioners, folk medicine sometimes with women. Green (1986) notes that electrical treatment was a "popular alternative" to traditional medicine in the 1870s in America (as well as a mainstream endeavor), sometimes administered by women. A "Mrs. French" delivered popular lectures on electrotherapeutics in Rochester, New York, in 1875, where "Mrs. Greenleaf" had an electrical practice for more than 25 years. Mrs. Greenleaf was listed as a "medical electrician" in the 1880 Rochester City Directory (Green, 1986: 167–169). Other female M.D.s also worked as electrotherapists and authors, including Emma Harding Britten, who published a book on *The Electrical Physician: Self-Cure Through Electricity* (1875).

Mary Putnam Jacobi published her *Essays on Hysteria, Brain Tumor and Some Other Cases of Nervous Diseases* in 1888. Perhaps the most famous female electrical physician in her own time was Margaret Cleaves, who wrote articles for several medical journals and authored a book on her own battle with mental illness, *The Autobiography of a Neurasthene: As Told by One of Them* (1910).

Despite continuing boundary disputes between legitimacy and quackery, mainstream and folk, however, the "Siamese twins" (Beard, 1874: 120) of neurology and electricity enjoyed considerable success in Victorian America (and England). Charles Dana, sketching the early history of neurology in the United States, recalled that when he received his first "combined galvanic and faradic battery" he "became the envy of the other clinicians who had no other tools but stethoscopes" (Dana, 1928: 1421). Neurology ultimately gave electricity a status above that of quackery; once officially sanctioned, electrical treatments for mental illness flourished until the first decade of the twentieth century.

"ELECTRICITY IS ALWAYS USEFUL"

The publication of Beard and Rockwell's *A Practical Treatise on the Medical and Surgical Uses of Electricity* (1867) marks the legitimation of electricity in treating mental illness in America. This book went through ten American editions and became a standard reference for electrotherapists, especially those treating nervous and mental disease. From his office in Lower Manhattan, George Beard, together with his partner Alphonse David Rockwell, defined the field (Rosenberg, 1962: 245–259; Rockwell, 1920: 182). Beard had used an induction coil to treat his own indigestion and nervousness while at Yale, and became interested in the efficacy of electricity. Working in the most competitive market for physicians in the United States, Beard found the possibility of a steady income from electrical treatment attractive. Unable to learn electrotherapeutics from established physicians such as Austin Flint, Beard became the protégé of Dr William Miller. Miller received $1.00 for each electrification and performed 25–30 per day, while the initially less experienced Beard charged half as much but made more than $400 his first year. Beard became the "Dean of American Electrotherapeutics" by altering the public and professional opinion of electrotherapy. As Rockwell later remembered: "Medical journals seldom referred to it [electrotherapy] in any way . . . with the exception of Garrat's ponderous and unphilosophical work. It was impossible to obtain any form of apparatus for the generation of a galvanic current, and all our earlier efforts in this direction were made with the inconsistent, inconvenient and ill smelling voltaic pile" (Rockwell, 1920: 193). Julius Althuis concurred, writing in the Preface to his 1870 *Treatise on Medical Electricity* that "ten years ago, medical men held galvanism in very low estimation; reports of cures by electricity were received with incredulous smiles" (p. 1).

But during the heyday of electrotherapeutics, Beard published and made money, and he was not the only one to do so. William Hammond, the United States surgeon general from 1862 to 1864, who was the first person to hold a chair in nervous and mental diseases in the United States, used this position to bring European electrotherapeutic works to the attention of American neurologists. Although they disagreed about many aspects of neurology, Hammond and Beard agreed that in cases of insanity "electricity is always useful" (Hammond, 1871: 394).

A group composed of neurologists, gynecologists, and general practitioners attempted to organize electrotherapeutics into an independent medical specialty. New York City neurologist William James Morton, professor of diseases of the mind and nervous system and electrotherapeutics at New York Post Graduate Medical school and editor of the *Journal of Nervous and Mental Diseases*, promoted the use of electrotherapy in mental illness. Morton, who had studied with Charcot in Paris, was instrumental in the formation of the New York Electrotherapeutic Society in 1883, and, together with neurologist William James Herdman and gynecologist George Betton Massey, formed a national association of electrotherapists. This group, the American Electrotherapeutical Association, played an active role in promoting electrotherapy. Its lecture series at the Columbian Exposition in 1893 proved so popular the group was forced to turn some members of the public away. President McKinley hosted them when they met in Washington in 1899, and they continued to draw large audiences at the International Exposition, held in St. Louis in 1904 (Nelson, 1993).

Electrotherapy was adopted in the curricula of some medical schools, and an 1894 survey of 140 deans of American medical colleges indicated that 80 out of the 90 respondents offered instruction in medical electricity. Institutions were created specifically to teach electrotherapy. The Electropathic Institute of Philadelphia applied for a charter to grant a doctorate of electrotherapeutics. A National College of Electrotherapeutics was established in Lima, Ohio in 1896, and electrotherapy could be learned from the International Correspondence School (ICS) (International Correspondence School, 1903). The *Journal of Electro-Therapeutics* was founded in 1890, later to become the *Journal of Advanced Therapeutics*, and, tellingly, in 1916, *The American Journal of Electrotherapeutics and Radiology* (Snow, 1925). For in the end—and despite their considerable success during the period 1870 to 1915—nineteenth-century electrotherapists were unable to create an independent medical specialty comparable to neurology or (later) radiology, remaining poised between the legitimate specialty of neurology on the one hand, and the specter of quackery on the other.

NEURASTHENIA, HYSTERIA, AND ELECTRICITY

The ancient association between electrical treatment and female hysteria continued into the nineteenth century, together with such disorders as chlorosis, chorea, brain fag, spinal irritation, and, above all, neurasthenia. Beard popularized (although he did not invent) neurasthenia, which, like ancient hysteria, was characterized by diffuse and sometimes mystifying symptoms including insomnia, forgetfulness, headaches, vertigo, and ringing in the ears (Beard, 1869: 217–221). By the end of the century, neurasthenia had become, in the medical and popular imagination, "alarmingly frequent," striking as many as "five million people of all ages" (Monell, 1910: 332). Beard set the stage for the electrical treatment of neurasthenic women and men.

Electrical treatment for neurasthenia incorporated galvanic, faradic, or static electricity, applied to the entire body, head, spine, or genitalia. Although originally a diagnosis related to the overwork or underwork of upper-middle-class males, within a short time these parameters changed. In response to diagnosing neurasthenia among women and lower-class men as well as among wealthy men, Beard and Rockwell proposed three subtypes of neurasthenia fitted to different social roles: "spinal neurasthenia (caused by physical labor or women's work), cerebrasthenic neurasthenia (caused by mental activity), and lithemic neurasthenia or autointoxication (caused by overindulgence)" (Cushing, 1995: 435). Other subtypes proposed by diagnosticians included cerebral neurasthenia, spinal neurasthenia, and sexual neurasthenia (Dana, 1925: 546; Schweig, 1879: 715; Beard, 1874: 438–451).

As in the eighteenth century, the temper of the times was among the proposed causes of neurasthenia. In 1900, one textbook claimed that neurasthenia was caused by daily and business cares, and that "many people" became "somewhat neurasthenic" at times (Jones, 1900: 323–334). Urbanization and its attendant wealth and stimulation were seen by Beard as a "predisposing" cause of neurasthenia, while sexual excess was among its "secondary" causes: "evil habits, excesses, tobacco, alcohol, worry, and special excitements, even climate itself . . . all the familiar excitants being secondary to the one great predisposing cause—civilization" (1881: 15). Both men and women were at risk here, women for their greater vulnerability to civilization, men for their greater temptations into "evil habits."

During the nineteenth century, electricity, gender, and sexuality were intertwined with the diagnosis and treatment of insanity. The ancient diagnosis of hysteria, with its gendered and sexualized implications, continued alongside that of neurasthenia. Both diagnoses were associated mainly with women—with their more vulnerable reproductive and nervous systems—but also, at times, with men (see Micale, 1991; Libbrecht and Quackelbush, 1995). By the time neurasthenia disappeared from the psychiatric vocabulary during the twentieth century, it had become known, like hysteria, as a diagnosis applied to women's troubles, although, as Micale (1991: 202) points out, roughly half of Beard's patients diagnosed with neurasthenia were men. Despite the diagnoses of male hysteria, the uterine female hysteria tradition survived the nineteenth century in "text after text" (King, 1993), some proposing uterine causation, and some not. Weir-Mitchell, for example, theorized that "irritations" of the reproductive system were transmitted electrically via nerve impulses to the brain (Vertinsky, 1990: 212). Such associations were criticized early in the century by Dewees, who wrote:

We would ask, then, what evidence is there, that the uterus possesses such unlimited sway over the healthy and diseased movements of almost every other portion of the body? Does not this error proceed from the influence of authority, and a supineness and indifference to rational inquiry and correct observation? Should the names of Hippocrates, Galen, Aretaeus, Van Helmont, and a hundred others of greater or less authority, be permitted so as to satisfy the judgment, or so paralyze exertion, as to prevent all investigation? (1828: 25)

Nonetheless, even in the latter part of the nineteenth century American medical handbooks continued to reflect uterine themes in the discussion of hysteria. At midcentury, Dr. Meigs, while concluding that female hysteria had multiple causes including the social, proposed that auras and vapors from the "diseased womb" rose to pervade other organs (1851: 479). For Meigs, female hysteria and electricity were isomorphic: "The hysterical woman, like the highly electrified thunder cloud, requires but the point to draw the flash" (1851: 488). Samuel Ashwell referred to the cure for hysteria as "women married happily and at a sufficiently early age becoming mothers" (1848: 172). In *Our Family Physician*, published in 1889, Dr. H.R. Stuart insisted that hypochondria and hysteria were afflictions of the mind, not, as in "ancient times," of the womb. Nevertheless, Dr. Stuart indicated that laces, heat, luxurious living, and violent emotions were to blame for female hysteria; the symptoms (throat strangulations) were almost exclusively the provenance of the widowed and unmarried, while the hysterical paroxysm was associated with the time of the menses (pp. 90–91).

Wrestling, similarly, with the problematics of uterus, mind, and social role in the etiology of hysteria, George Napheys noted that hysteria and mania were "almost exclusively confined to single persons" (1875: 386). The curative powers of marriage for women existed, as they had for millennia, but they were located in the social and not the reproductive order: "Marriage exerts a decidedly curative influence" because "Success . . . is always a tonic. . . . Now to women, marriage is a success. It is their aim in social life; and this accomplished, health and strength follow" (pp. 386–387). Nevertheless, Napheys returned to the uterine theme at other points in his text. He referred to menopause as a time when the woman is "finishing her pilgrimage of sexual life" and "shades of moral insanity" appear; she must curb any sexual desires she has since this is "contrary to nature" (Napheys, 1875: 392–402). Among the many treatments proposed by nineteenth-century physicians for hysteria were electrical and Galen's widow's treatments—sometimes separately, sometimes in combination.

THE WOMAN ON THE COUCH: GENDER, SEXUALITY, AND ELECTRICAL TREATMENT

Counterpointed to the pauper lunatic in the asylum as the canonical nineteenth-century patient is the upper-middle-class woman on the couch (Jordanova, 1989), reclining at the behest of the moral, electrical, or psychoanalytical physician. Among the repertoire of the electrical physician was, as it had been for two thousand years, the genital treatment of insanity; by the nineteenth century, Galen's widow's treatment (see the Preface) had not disappeared, it had merely gone underground. Because of the reticence of Victorian writers concerning the topic of sexuality it is difficult to draw our own textual boundary between anachronistic prurience and head-in-the-sand denial. Victorian physicians, if they wrote at all about the sexual meanings of electrical treatments, wrote about the patients, not themselves. One rare exception was Dr. Beck, who deliberately induced an orgasm in a woman patient and then questioned her about her sensations, saying, "Here then was an opportunity never before offered any one to my knowledge, and not to be lost on any consideration" (Flint, 1874: 338).

Contemporary secondary sources point the sexualized finger at some nineteenth-century physicians. It is hard for us, for example, not to read eroticism into the following account, from an 1848 issue of the "phreno-mesmeric" journal *The Zoist*. A Miss Aglonby, of the Nunnery in Cumberland, reported that her mesmerist, "Mr. Nixon," had sent her into a trance while applying galvanic shocks. In the first treatment, on June 7, "Mr. Nixon retreated a few steps from me . . . I felt drawn irresistibly to him as the needle by the magnet." On June 16, "My mesmeriser, by taking my aunt by the hand, placed her *en rapport* with me; but here some cross-mesmerism seemed to take place, for I felt confused, and alternately repelled from and attracted to both." The next day after a treatment, she was left "mesmerised and lying on the sofa with the organ of language excited." Nixon returned within 30 minutes, "but, some minutes before he arrived, I felt a glow of warmth with a perspiration all over me, and my breathing became quick, panting, and difficult." During these sessions, Mr. Nixon "stimulated . . . points" in Miss Aglonby's body corresponding to phrenological categories such as Veneration, Imagination, and Imitation (1848: 238–240).

Taylor (1983) describes Beard and Rockwell's electrical techniques as a fusion of the sexual body of the patient with the sexual body of the physician, through the transfer of electricity from one to the other. During the procedure, Taylor writes, both male and female patients removed all their "upper" clothing, females "covering themselves modestly with a sheet." The patient's feet were placed on a copper plate, the negative pole of the electrical charge. The operator held the positive electrode, wrapped in a sponge, in his hand, squeezing and releasing the sponge to vary the current. The current passed through the operator's body (bulking up his arm muscles over time) and transferred through his "slightly moistened" hand to the patient's spine, muscles, and "entire body." Taylor suggests that the operator "experienced the same exhilaration and tonic effects from the current passing through their bodies as did the patients" (Taylor, 1983: 282).

Beard and Rockwell's descriptions of their treatment procedures, often using the electric hand, echo the body parts of the widow treated by Galen, but not the orgasmic or pleasurable response. In a typical case of "hysteria, in the person of a married lady aged 40," the treatment consisted of "thorough general faradization, and immediately after a galvanic current from eight cells was nearly as possible located in the uterus. These efforts were followed by decided alleviation of the symptoms" (Beard and Rockwell, 1888: 422). Beard and Rockwell's treatments for hysteria were often related to the reproductive system and menstrual cycle. Of the six cases of female hysteria "and allied afflictions" recounted in their 1881 textbook, one involved suppressed menstruation, one pregnancy, one postpartum depression, one excessive menstruation, and one "menopause insanity in a married lady" (1881: 440).

Local, genital electrical, or other stimulatory treatments for female hysteria were subject to debate among Victorian physicians, as they had been among Renaissance theologians (Schleiner, 1991; Maines, 1999). The invention of the speculum for internal genital examinations, and (later in the century) of anesthesia, gave impetus to the burgeoning discipline of gynecology. However, both spectacular examinations and genital surgery were considered highly improper by some practitioners, the one likely to over-sex, and the other to un-sex the female patient. Lee Benjamin, writing in 1891, warned that "Manipulating" the female reproductive organs "directly through the vagina, as recommended by Reeves Jackson and others, is not sufficient to counterbalance the serious objections to the procedure on the score of delicacy and the risk of inducing involuntary erotic manifestations on the part of the patient" (pp. 332–333). Other practitioners disavowed internal examination, but allowed external genital stimulation, possibly on the ancient grounds that only penetration constituted "real" sex (Mitchison, 1991). In 1906 Neiswanger commented that electrical "Vibration . . . causes sexual emotions" (p. 244). He warned that "The employment of vibratory stimulation *within* the rectum, urethra, or female pelvis cannot be too strongly condemned, although in many instances it may be used upon the *outside* for relief of pelvic disturbances" (Neiswanger, 1906: 241; see also Eberhart, 1913).

Following the ancient Hippocratic and Galenic pathways to the treatment of hysteria, some nineteenth-century American and European physicians used both desexing and resexing local treatments. Desexing treatments included ovariotamy or (sometimes galvanoelectrical) clitoridectomy (see Scull and

Favreau, 1981; Ripa, 1990; Longo, 1979), while treatments that might be seen by we moderns as sexualizing included the electrical stimulation of the female (and at times male) genitalia. McGinnis, for example, noted that electricity was "of service" in the removal of the overdeveloped clitoris that "interfered with marital intercourse" (1894: 2). By contrast, Ashwell recommended the galvanic treatment of hysteria combined with amenorrhea, since "the paroxysm and its immediate results have been materially relieved" (1848: 177), while Tripier referred to a faradic attachment as "the uterine exciter" (1884: 140). These genital techniques of treating women's insanity, including clitoridectomy, continued into the early decades of the twentieth century (King, 1901; Hedley, 1900; Taylor, 1905; Reynolds, 1910; Paramore, 1921; Diefendorf, 1923; Maines, 1999). Robert Taylor, a professor at Columbia University, recommended, in 1905, "full excision of the clitoris" for "some" cases of "nymphomania" (Taylor, 1905: 422).

Other physicians were less sanguine about the genital treatment of hysteria or other mental disorders. Dr. Zenner of Philadelphia warned against "the frequent inutility or needlessness of local treatment" of hysteria (1883: 523–524). He himself had tried both ovariotomy and an introduced pessary with his patients, neither of which had been successful. Zenner regarded genital interventions into female insanity as causing, rather than curing, mental and sexual symptoms, warning of patients' "delusions or hallucinations of a sexual type, in which the examining physician was a central figure" (Zenner, 1883: 525). From the other side of the Atlantic, Dr. Clifford Allbutt, fellow of the Royal College of Physicians, concurred with Zenner's (1883: 523) depiction of gynecological interventions as, by the 1880s, "only too fashionable":

A neuralgic woman seems . . . to be particularly unfortunate . . . she is either told that she is hysterical or that it is all uterus . . . in the second case she is entangled in the net of the gynaecologist, who finds her uterus, like her nose, is a little on one side, or again, like that organ, is running a little, or it is as flabby as her biceps, so that the unhappy viscus is impaled upon a stem, or perched upon a prop, or painted with carbolic acid every week in the year except during the long vacation when the gynaecologist is grouse-shooting, or salmon-catching, or leading the fashion in the Upper Engadine. (1884: 17)

Early twentieth-century physicians continued to criticize genital treatments for female insanity. Reynolds warned that "with intractable neurotics, local treatment, whether operative or minor, usually only fixes the attention of the patient and increases the evil" (1910: 113). Paramore cited the case of a 29-year-old woman treated vaginally with a pessary for neurasthenia: she was operated upon and subsequently became worse, diagnosed with melancholia (1921: 116). In 1923, Diefendorf suggested that the surgical removal of healthy ovaries for hysteria should be "discarded today," although pressure "upon the hysterogenic zones" and "simple suggestion" might be useful.

Electrical physicians in the nineteenth century were concerned with the control of male as well as female sexual behavior in the name of mental health, including "masturbatory insanity." In 1898, Beard published *Sexual Neurasthenia*, summarizing his work to date on the causes and treatment of this disorder. In this book electricity is described as "the most important and efficient remedy among a long list" of treatments for sexual neurasthenia (p. 224). Overindulgence in intercourse, or masturbation, led to exhaustion and impotence in men, which "electricity revives" (Beard, 1898: 232–233; see also Erb, 1883: 252). Hysteria, as well as neurasthenia, was sometimes linked with men and with male sexuality. Charcot, famous in France for his performing female hysterics, also treated male hysterics, first at the Bicetre and from 1882 in a new Salpetrière "Service des Hommes" (Micale, 1991: 203). Jewell and Bannister's (1874) study of 38 cases of hysteria must have included at least half men, since they found electrical treatment effective with "nineteen cases of pollution and impotence" (p. 325). Meigs, in a case history of male hysteria, claimed that hysterical men had "frequent erections" as well as "globus," and suffered the "morbid aphrodisiac element of unrequited love" (1851: 480–481). Other aspects of hierarchy than gender and sex, including occupation and race, were implicated in nineteenth-century psychiatric theorizing and electrical treatment. Dr. George Schweig reported in 1877 that the neurasthenics he had treated with electric baths included two overworked male lawyers and one underoccupied gentleman of leisure (pp. 85–90). His one melancholic case was a butcher, while his two hysterical married women were reported, respectively, as "sterile" and as suffering from postpartum symptoms (Schweig, 1877: 83–84, 122–123); an excellent example of the era's gendered Catch-22.

There are a number of case histories from the late eighteenth to the early twentieth centuries describing the local, genital electrical treatment of male pollution, impotence, nocturnal emissions, homosexuality, masturbation, or other "inappropriate" spending or hoarding of male semen. Tipton (1882) equated the etiologies and treatments of nymphomania and spermatorrhea. He suggested putting a pint or so of water in a mug, and putting the penis and testicles in it with the positive electrode, while moving the negative electrode with a long cord, "over the lumbar vertebrae. . . . If a female a sponge roll may be placed between the labia. . . . Otherwise treat the same as males" (pp. 150–151). Similarly, de Watteville noted that "I have frequently had the opportunity in the outpatients' room to observe the beneficial effect of the current on the penis and sense of weariness or discomfort . . . [as with] various ovarian or uterine derangements" (1884: 196).

Yet despite the presence of men in the domains of neurasthenia, hysteria, and electricity—as well as the lunatic asylum—the woman on the couch remains the central image of nineteenth-century psychiatric practice, evoking a multitude of associations, from Charlotte Perkins Gilman's "Yellow Wallpaper" to Sigmund Freud's talking cure (Jordanova, 1989). It is an upper-class image, reflecting women, such as Alice James and Virginia Woolf, who neglected their reproductive system in favor of their intellectual development, and thus brought about neurasthenic or hysterical symptoms. In the 1870s, Naphey concluded that hysteria was common in puberty, especially in "those higher circles of society, where their emotions are over-educated and their organization delicate" (1875: 38). Electricity was used to treat these women not only by electrotherapists such as Beard, but also by those who engaged in rival approaches—moral treatment and psychoanalysis.

Moral treatment for hysteria and neurasthenia was indicated for the languishing, unmarried, or unsettled married upper-class woman during the nineteenth century, and electricity was one of the ways in which the body of the morally treated woman was stimulated during her long incarceration. In his book *Fat and Blood* (1877) Weir Mitchell described moral treatment as "a combination of entire rest and of excessive feeding, made possible by passive exercise obtained through steady use of massage and electricity" (p. 7). Mitchell's theory of disease was not uterine, but in practice most of his patients were female because he "believed that males would not tolerate the enforced idleness he required" (Wood, 1973: 38).

According to Wood (1973: 31), the women treated by Weir Mitchell were massaged and electrically vibrated for an hour a day, as they lay passively in bed. Wood suggests that Weir Mitchell combined electrical vibration with mesmeric powers, rendering his moral treatment highly sexualized—he threatened to undress and get into bed with one "recalcitrant" patient (1973: 39). In claiming for himself and other male physicians the patriarchal power of a father, or god, he "skated on the edge of primitive healing through mesmeric sexual powers" (1973: 38). The same kind of criticism has often been leveled at Sigmund Freud, the patriarch of the psychoanalytic couch.

Freud was led to his couch, and "Breuer's talking cure" (Taylor, 1983: 282) by failures of electrical treatment. Early in his career, Freud used "brief shocks to the back and limbs" to treat neurasthenics (Alverno, 1990: 54), a procedure he found useless. Eventually, "I put my electrical apparatus aside, even before Mobius had solved the problem by explaining that the successes of electrical treatment in nervous disorders (insofar as there were any) were the effect of suggestion on the part of the physician" (Freud, 1952: 28). Under the combined weight of the talking cure and of the direct sale of electrotherapeutic devices through catalogs, physicians' use of electrotherapeutics for mental disorder waned during the first part of the twentieth century.

ELECTROTHERAPEUTICS AND THE MARKETPLACE

At the turn of the century, electricity was well established in the arsenal of medicine. It appeared to provide relief or cure for a number of ailments:

cataphoresis, rheumatism, hysterical paralysis, infantile paralysis (polio), neuralgia, uterine or vaginal disorders, chorea, hysteria, neurasthenia, and some other classifications of insanity (Haller, 1971: 1142; Sajous, 1925: 13). But during the first decade of the twentieth century, reclassifications of mental diseases, and alterations in the profession of neurology, began to unravel the link between electrical treatment and disorders such as neurasthenia and hysteria.

While the heyday of public interest in electricity and electrotherapy was from about 1870 to 1915, there were some earlier indications of a professional turn away from the use of electrotherapy. The membership of the American Electro-Therapeutic Association declined from a peak of 280 to 225 in 1915 (*World Almanac*, 1915: 563). After years of attempts, there was still no standard nomenclature for electrical treatment, and treatments were not widely accepted (De Kraft, 1917: 5–13). A survey of the *American Journal of Insanity* revealed little interest in electricity, much interest in drug therapy, and some hostility among alienists to practitioners of electrical medicine such as George Beard (Everts, 1880). Although the work of both Weir Mitchell and Freud was based in part in electricity, the psychological elements became more significant, as practitioners employed moral and psychoanalytic treatment, rather than the somatic. The mental hygiene and religious "mind-cure" movements also played a part in the early twentieth-century turn away from somaticism and toward the mind as a source of both the cause and cure of mental illness (Kneeland, 1996).

The dominant etiology and modality of treatment for mental disorder in America became, during the early decades of the twentieth century, the psychoanalytical, and especially the Freudian. The dominance of this model during and after the world wars is evident from the proliferation of psychoanalytic societies during the period from 1911–1941 (Bunker, 1944: 495; Hale, 1995). Psychoanalysis also influenced physicians in the hospitals located in and around New York City (Burnham, 1967: 156–158). The psychoanalytical framework informed what one historian has labeled the "psychiatric persuasion" of the years between World War I and II (Lunbeck, 1984). Beginning at leading institutes such as the Boston Psychopathic Hospital, the Phipps Clinic, and the New York Neurological Clinic, psychiatrists utilizing the theory of unconscious extended the span of their discipline beyond the realm of the insane and over virtually everyone else as well. By abandoning a fixed dichotomy between normal and abnormal, psychiatrists suggested that the entire population suffered from some kind of mental ill health; the rise of psychological testing classification and quantification provided an empirical basis for these claims (Lasch, 1979). Under the new paradigm, disorders such as hysteria and neurasthenia were reexamined and a psychological rather than a somatic etiology was proclaimed (Sicherman, 1977; Dana, 1904). Neurology, once twinned with electricity, followed new intellectual paths, including social learning theory and psychoanalysis; some neurologists even came to believe that the effects of electricity were psychological (Tilney, 1924: 57).

During and after World War I, a number of institutions once receptive to medical electricity, such as the University of Pennsylvania and Harvard University, dropped electrotherapeutics and moved electric treatments into departments of physiotherapy (Granger, 1920: 448). Although some "shell shocked" soldiers were treated with electricity, the United States Army decided not to adopt electrotherapeutics as an independent treatment modality in its 38 hospitals (Snow, 1925: 115). National and state medical associations rejected papers on electrotherapy, or allowed them only into sections of physiotherapy (Snow, 1923: 31–32). The rise of third-party payers after World War I also played a part in the derailing of electrotherapeutics as a medical specialty. Insurance companies did not recognize electrotherapy apart from neurology or orthopedics; therefore they would only pay for electrical physiotherapy (Snow, 1923: 33).

Electricity moved, between the world wars, from general practice to physiotherapy and radiology. Both the *Alienist and Neurologist* and the *Medical Record* ceased publication after World War I, leaving only the *American Journal of Electrotherapeutics and Radiology* to serve as an outlet for publications on electrical treatment. However, in 1924 even this journal changed its name to reflect a new emphasis on the growing area of physical therapy: the *Physical Therapeutics* (Kovacs, 1925: 313–316). In 1929 the American Electrotherapeutic Association merged with the Western Association of Physical Therapy to form the American Physical Therapy Association (Kovacs, 1925: 18). Once electrotherapy was reclassified as a physical therapy, the use of electricity to treat mental disorder began to decline.

The public perception of electricity also changed between the wars from one of positive utopia, to domesticity on the one hand, and danger on the other. After the turn of the century, nearly every daily task changed as electricity became commonplace. But the transition from decentralized batteries to centralized alternating current could also be deadly. On October 31 1917, Dr. Arthur M. Clapp died "while adjusting or testing a new high frequency apparatus" which he had connected to the main power from the street. "He was found in the doorway leading from the waiting room to the inner office, both hands connected to the circuit, which was running at full power" (obituary, 1917). Thomas Edison, who had engendered fantastic hopes and fears about the powers of electricity, was, along with A.D. Rockwell, associated with the invention of the electric chair (Nye, 1991: 253). Despite a general decline, electrotherapeutics lingered on in a variety of private sanitaria, as advertisements in the *Journal of Nervous and Mental Disease* showed. Recommendations for nervous exhaustion, mild neuroses, and nervous headaches included galvanic and static treatment (Kovacs, 1932: 118), while some practitioners treated mental symptoms with faradization (King, 1901; Showalter, 1985: 166–167) or static electricity (Metcalfe, 1911). Faithful adherents of electrotherapy for mental illness, such as William Benham Snow, continued to insist that neurasthenia and hysteria were organic illnesses and best treated by electricity (1922: 60–61). The passing of Snow and his generation ended the first widespread and systematic modern use of electricity and allowed a sort of historical amnesia to develop surrounding the early uses of electrotherapy.

But there was one locale in which electrotherapeutics flourished during the late nineteenth and early twentieth centuries in America: the marketplace. This era saw a vast expansion of the capitalist marketplace, including the direct market for electrical devices found in catalog sales. Alongside electrical household items such as hair curlers or mixers, these catalogs sold electrical and magnetic devices or potions aimed at the self-diagnosis and cure of illness—bypassing the physician altogether, and liable to charges of quackery by him. One such direct-marketed item, a medicine said to contain "liquid electricity," was patented by Thomas Edison in 1879 and remained on the market for many years. By ingesting electricity, the patient would "commingle with it, and draw upon its power. It was a magical fluid, a nerve-tingling juice" (Nye, 1991: 153–155). Other items for sale included electrical (and magnetic) devices for the relief of various physical, nervous, and mental symptoms. "Addison's galvanic" electric belts were marketed as "Nature's Vitalizer," and condemned in an AMA series on *Nostrums and Quackery* first published in 1912. "Nolan's Famous Catarrh Cure," banned by the U.S. Post Office in 1930, promised to deliver "50,000 volts of electricity in a two drachm bottle" (Armstrong and Armstrong, 1991: 191–193). As in all eras before and since, the physician's response to direct-marketing of therapeutics was rarely positive. In the words of Henry Tibbets, who treated both male and female genitalia with electricity:

the medical practitioner who prescribes electricity should either administer it himself, or cause it to be administered by a skilled operator . . . when patients themselves apply electricity, the result has been very unsatisfactory. The most explicit directions will often be misunderstood, or fail in being correctly carried out, the treatment getting undeserved discredit. The rule of practice here laid down is particularly applicable to the local application of electricity. (1873: 160)

Some of the advertisements for these devices appealed to the general reader, like Thomas Edison's electrical juice. A 1910 brain galvanization machine, for example, promised the cure of various disorders including neurasthenia, and even posed advantages to the physician: "The machine can be without fear given into the hands of the ill person, to whom can be given a fast and easy instruction in the mode of employment; a great saving of time for the doctor." Other advertisements were gendered or even sexualized in their appeal, restoring domesticity to the housewife or sexuality to the male head of household—and both to their respective work roles. In 1892, in a testimonial-advertising letter, a "prostrate" "young married wife of six months" who had "kept house for only four months" before her "nervous breakdown" was "Snatched from Death and the Grave, a young wife restored to her loving husband and good friends in good health" by an electric belt. By contrast, the $18 Giant Power Heidelberg Electric Belt advertised in a 1901 Sears catalog was aimed at "those sexually weak or impotent or suffering from any trouble of the sexual organs. . . . The stimulating alternating current forces a vigorous circulation of blood into the seminal glands, enlivening them into a healthy glow. . . . The 80-gauge current absolutely doubles the sexual force and power." Although there were advertisements for vibrators aimed at women in these *fin de siècle* catalogs, any sexualized references were indirect, relying on allusions such as "thrilling, invigorating, penetrating, revitalizing . . . living pulsing touch" (Maines, 1989: 7–9). Galen's widow's treatment had left the field of medicine and entered the modern household (Maines, 1999).

After World War I the electrotherapist faced challenges from psychoanalysis and from the direct marketing of electrical devices—and retired for a time from the public arena. In 1929, the fourteenth edition of the *Encyclopædia Britannica* closed a chapter in the history of electrotherapeutics by declaring that it was "a general term for electricity in the alleviation and cure of disease. Many claims have been made for its use in the past which could not be justified, or were at best psychological" (Pring, 1929: 342–343). It was practically an obituary; but it turned out to be a premature one.

PART II

THE ELECTROCONVULSIVE CENTURY

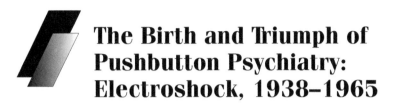

Chapter 3

The Birth and Triumph of Pushbutton Psychiatry: Electroshock, 1938–1965

[The psychiatrist] is now ridiculed because of his propensity to treat certain of his patients with a gadget—an electroshock machine! He is now referred to as an "electrician" and a "push button practitioner" and other opprobrious and less printable terms.

—Gilbert Adamson, 1955

In the mid-twentieth century in America, electricity combined with convulsion in electroshock. Originating in the same Mediterranean region that had nurtured the uses of amber and the electric eel, electroshock came to dominate the repertoire of European and American somatic therapies for mental disease. And, despite professional, legal and lay challenges to the treatment during the decades of the 1960s–1980s (see Chapter 4), the use of electroshock continued throughout the twentieth century and into the new millennium (see Chapter 5).

EST is a treatment that brings together the head and brain of the patient with the electrical machine. Electrodes are placed on the patient's head either unilaterally (one electrode) or bilaterally (two, generally on the temporal lobes but sometimes on the back and front of the head); an electrical current is passed through the brain, generating an epileptic seizure in the patient. While early EST treatments were generally bilateral, psychiatrists experimented with unilateral placement during the 1970s and 1980s, returning to bilateral placement (in many cases) by the late twentieth century (Pearlman, 1991: 132).

There were different types of electroshock developed during the 1940s–1960s in America and Europe, including glissando EST (Steinfeld, 1951), a method that incorporated a gradual rise in current flow from zero to preset coordinates (Impastato et al., 1957: 381), and Multiple-Monitored ECT (MMECT), in which multiple seizures rather than a single seizure are induced during the coma (Mielke et al., 1984). There was also regressive EST, described by Abrams (1986: 26) as "conducted at some American hospitals during the fifties. [It] entailed daily treatments. . . . So intensive a regimen rendered the patient profoundly disoriented, unable to speak or remember, incontinent . . . the therapy was based on the naive theory that if a neurotic patient regressed to an infantile state, his personality could be restructured by means of psychoanalytic techniques as he gradually returned to normal."

Early EST machines and treatments were simple, violent, and frequent, with unsedated patients receiving shocks as high as 190 volts, sometimes many times a week for several years, although some psychiatrists did sedate their patients (Steinfeld, 1951: 125). The technology of EST changed between the 1940s and the late 1990s, with (in theory at least) more closely calibrated and computerized machinery, lower voltages, shorter periods of electricity, and fewer treatments during one course of treatment. The introduction of various muscle relaxants or sedatives by the 1950s, and later general anesthesia recommended prior to EST, added the services of the anesthesiologist to the otherwise inexpensive procedure.

The context for the development and popularization of EST included the cyclical "crisis" of overpopulated mental hospitals, the predominance of somatic psychiatric theories of mental illness, and a wartime environment that encompassed both European fascism and the psychiatric hospitalization of American soldiers in areas around the Mediterranean. The new technology, originating in fascist Italy, soon spread to the democratic nations of Europe and America. And, as with previous electrical cures, American physicians who used EST organized into professional associations, started up journals, and published their success stories inside those journals.

EST flourished in America in an atmosphere of crisis; from the 1920s through the 1940s the media quoted psychiatrists alarmed at what they called a "health care crisis" in the treatment of the mentally ill. The public was told that the numbers of mentally ill were "increasing more rapidly than provisions are made for their care" (Hutchins, 1939: 3). In his presidential address before the American Psychiatric Association, Owen Copp claimed that "the number of beds for the treatment of mental disease in public institutions throughout the United States *equals, probably exceeds* the aggregate for all other forms of illness" (italics added, 1921: 22; see also Malzberg, 1943: 487–488). In 1948 the *New York Times* declared, "Mental illness will be spoken of as our number one problem in public health for an indefinite period of time." This editorial claimed that mental patients occupied 50 percent of all hospital beds, and that there was an "increase of 21 percent in the incidence of insanity in the American population from 1940–1945" ("New Horizons in Psychiatry," 3 January 1948: 12). A national census of state mental institutions indicated that institutionalized populations increased 16.3 percent from 1937–1946, while the number of first-time admissions to state hospitals rose from 78,000 to 89,000 (Felix, 1949: xi–xii).

Not only were more people than ever institutionalized in America, they were often permanently institutionalized (Grob, 1983: 12), and the conditions of their institutionalization were sometimes inhumane. One reporter saw "hundreds of naked mental patients herded into barnlike, filth-infested wards" where they were "shackled, strapped, strait-jacketed and bound to their beds" (Deutsch, 1948: 449). Another critic of institutions recalled how mental patients spent "weeks at a stretch" restrained by " 'muffs', 'miffs', wristlets, locks and straps," confined to lodges that at night became "black tombs in which the cries of the insane echo unheard from the peeling plaster of the walls" (Maisel, 1946: 103). Humanization of treatment for the mentally ill took several forms, including a switch from referring to institutions that care for the mentally ill as "asylums" to calling them "hospitals," and a search for cures, especially for those suffering from the severe psychotic and schizophrenic disorders.

Although popular, psychotherapy was not particularly helpful for the chronically mentally ill, many of whom were lower class, minorities, or immigrants. In response to psychotherapy's apparent failure among institutionalized populations, a number of biological theories and somatic treatments of mental illness were proposed. Psychiatrist Henry Cotton of the New Jersey Institute for Insanity commented that there had been a fourfold increase in the insane population at the same time as the practice of psychotherapy had become institutionalized in American psychiatry. He concluded "it is not giving away any secrets and not even an exaggeration to state that this method has been a complete failure" (Cotton, 1930: 57). Thus, by the 1930s, many psychiatrists working in the state hospitals had come to reject the "talking cure" in favor of somatic treatments.

THE RISE OF SOMATIC TREATMENTS

Somatic treatments for mental illness range from the most invasive procedures such as brain surgery, to the least invasive such as gentle hydrotherapy and mild pharmacology. Although somatic treatments are rarely absent from the repertoire of psychiatry, somatic therapy in general and specific treatments options rise and fall over time. During the period between World War I and II, interest in somatic therapy was high and a number of new somatic treatments developed: hydrotherapy (used in American mental hospitals into the 1970s), diathermy, or heat therapy (Rowbottom and Susskind, 1984: 195), brain surgery, and the convulsive therapies.

Somatic theories and treatments proliferated in Europe during the 1920s and 1930s, a time when eugenic theories in science and fascist eugenics in politics flourished in Europe and North America. One American state hospital report noted that between 1939 and 1941 it had sterilized six mental patients, then lamented: "It is unfortunate that we have been unable to sterilize more cases, particularly those who are at large. We must face the fact that the nation is being poisoned by the rapid production of mental and moral defectives, and to insure the survival of the fittest we have to abrogate defectives, of all power to procreate" (Delaware State Hospital, 1941: 22–23). The 1927 Nobel Prize in medicine went to Austrian Julius Wagner von Jauregg, whose fever therapy promised a new cure for psychosis. Jauregg injected his neuro-syphilitic patients with a variety of substances, such as tuberculin, typhus, and malaria; the attendant high fever seemed to reduce the symptoms of psychosis. Following the International Conference on Fever Therapy in New York City in 1937, fever therapy was disseminated throughout the United States, and was in widespread use until the late 1950s in the treatment of psychosis (Roback and Keirnan, 1969: 263).

During the 1930s, Manfred Sakel in Vienna and Ladislaus Meduna in Budapest began to treat schizophrenic patients with chemically induced convulsions (Rowbottom and Susskind, 1984: 193). Sakel accidentally produced an insulin coma in one of his patients and noted that the patient's psychotic symptoms abated; he named his new treatment *Insulinshockbehandlung*. Refined insulin shock consisted of giving the patient a daily injection of insulin, gradually increasing the dose until the patient lapsed into a coma. Patients were brought out of a coma through application of a glucose solution. Daily treatments of insulin/glucose could last weeks (Braslow, 1997: 97). Traveling to Wingsdale, New York in 1936, Sakel demonstrated his therapy to psychiatrists who disseminated it throughout the United States. In the mid-1950s Sakel claimed an 88 percent success rate in treating schizophrenia (Sakel, 1954: 255–316), and the treatment remained in use until the 1960s, although overshadowed by ECT (Sakel, 1938: 1–13; Barton, 1987: 164).

In Hungary, Meduna conducted a series of autopsies on the brains of epileptics and schizophrenics, concluding that schizophrenics had a less than normal amount of glia tissue while epileptics had more, and that epilepsy and schizophrenia were antagonistic to one another (Meduna, 1954: 215–222; Berrios, 1997: 108). In 1936 Meduna experimentally induced convulsions among patients diagnosed as schizophrenic using chemical agents such as pentylenetetrazol, also known as Metrazol or Cardazol (Grob, 1985: 104). As Europe moved toward World War II, both Sakel and Meduna emigrated to the United States where they helped popularize convulsive treatment.

Another somatic treatment in the battle against mental disorder was hydrotherapy. Hydrotherapy has a long history of its own, and was used in nineteenth-century asylums (Dent, 1903: 91). Treatment consisted of various techniques, including the continuous bath: restraining a patient in a canvas-covered bathtub filled with cold or hot water for anywhere from one to twelve hours. In another variation, attendants wrapped a patient in wet sheets or blankets for hours at a time. In the early 1940s hydrotherapy was "one of the most important departments" at East Moline State Hospital in Illinois, and lasted there into the 1960s (East Moline State Hospital 1963: 4–5, 64). However, like electrotherapy it was subsumed into physical therapy and was dropped as a stand-alone treatment for mental disorder.

Surgery has been among the most invasive somatic treatments of mental disease for centuries. In the United States Henry Cotton, believing that insanity was caused by autointoxication, surgically removed teeth (Cotton, 1930: 57) and the large bowel (Shorter, 1997: 112), claiming they were the source of the "focal infections" causing insanity. However the pre-eminent surgery for mental illness from 1930 to 1960 was prefrontal lobotomy or leucotomy, pioneered by Egaz Moniz Portugal. Moniz drilled two holes in the cranium to remove all or part of the prefrontal lobes (Pressman, 1998: 52–54; Swayze, 1995: 505–518). After the procedure, once violent and uncontrolled patients, the majority of whom were women and children, were said to become tractable and malleable. Moniz received a Nobel Prize for his brain surgery for insanity. In the United States Walter Freeman and James Watts pioneered the treatment of the insane with lobotomy, and there were perhaps 25,000 such treatments performed between 1936 and 1953 (Freeman, 1953: 70). Duin and Sutcliffe (1992: 119) note that lobotomy, as an even more invasive treatment than ECT, "became standard in patients resistant to shock therapy."

Somatic treatments for the chronically mentally ill were adopted in the United States during the 1930s and 1940s in an era of perceived mental health crisis and a turn toward biological explanations for mental disease. Somatic experimentation involved health risks. Metrazol convulsions sometimes caused broken teeth and bone fractures, while insulin shock could lead to pulmonary edema and a mortality rate of between 1 percent and 2 percent (Braslow, 1997: 97). Still, the alternative of doing nothing was unpalatable to the physicians at the time, who referred to abandoning people to the "living death of mental disease" (Van De Water, 1940). Thus, the search for new and safer forms of convulsive therapy paved the way for electrical and chemical convulsive treatment in American psychiatry.

THE BIRTH OF ELECTROSHOCK: ROME, APRIL 15, 1938

The only somatic treatment developed in the 1930s still widely available today is electroshock. Although most "origin myths" concerning ECT focus on the 1930s, there are proposals in the literature for earlier precedents, including the ancient Roman use of electric eels (see the Preface; and Harms, 1955: 933). Alexander and Selesnick (1966: 394) claim that "probably the first electroconvulsive treatment for mental illness was administered by a French physician, J.B. LeRoy, in 1775, on a patient with psychogenic blindness," and that Swiss physician Michael Shuppach "applied it [electroshock] successfully some two hundred years" before the 1938 "invention" of ECT by Cerletti and Bini (p. 56). In 1837, Dr. John Armstrong told this story:

I knew a gentleman who desired a medical man to send him some medicine to take, "for he had seven devils." The doctor said he did not like to take any man's word upon such a subject, and wished to investigate the case personally. He called on his patient, and having examined him said, "Seven devils! You have eight, and the eighth is worse than all the others put together." It was agreed between them that the doctor should adopt some means of driving out these devils; and the first was accordingly driven out by a slight electric shock, and the others in succession by shocks increasing in power, till only the eighth devil remained; and then the doctor, to git [*sic*] rid of this troublesome guest took care that the shock should be strong enough to knock the patient down and he was cured. (Armstrong, 1837: 313–314)

These early prototypes of electroshock continued into the early twentieth century. By World War I, according to Rowbottom and Susskind (1984: 192–193), "experimental induction of epileptic convulsions by means of an electric shock became a recognized physiological procedure."

Rome was the site of Ugo Cerletti's quest for new psychiatric treatments; there in the mid-1930s he led a team of medical researchers consisting of Lucio Bini, Ferdinando Accornero, and Mario Felici (Shorter, 1997: 218–219). Cerletti, who had visited Vienna to study the effects of insulin with Sakel, began work with his team on chemical forms of convulsion which were abandoned after their eventual "discovery" of electroshock (Kalinowsky, 1980: 430). The research, funded by and conducted during the Italian Fascist movement, formed part of broader efforts of a variety of experts in medicine and social science to assume the role of social managers and engineers. These experts sought ways to ameliorate the perceived social pathologies that plagued modern Italy. One fascist spokesman lamented the price of such pathologies: "The State, agencies, and individuals pay harshly—in ever-growing costs of asylums, hospitals, sanitaria, prisons" (Horn, 1994: 43). Cerletti himself subscribed to a fascist magazine, and may have identified with the movement (Horn, 1994: 60–61).

Cerletti and Bini's experiment with EST was prompted by Cerletti's observation of the effect of electric stunning on hogs being readied for slaughter. After Bini discovered the means to induce nonfatal convulsions in dogs, the team abandoned their other research to pursue this approach, which Cerletti named electroshock (Berrios, 1997: 110). Many versions of the first electroshock exist, and the date of the first remains in dispute (Berrios, 1997: 110n) although everyone agrees that an electroshock event occurred in April 1938. Witnessing this event were Cerletti, Bini, Vittorio Calliol, Mario Felici, Spartaco Mazzanti, an aide, and Ferdinando Accornero, a clinic assistant (Accornero, 1988). Below is Alverno's version of the first electroshock:

One morning in April 1938, in total secrecy, the patient was taken to a remote room on the first floor of the institute. He was quite docile and lay quietly on the examining table. One assistant, Calliol, was guarding the door to chase away intruders. Cerletti, Bini, Felici, Accornero, and a male nurse were in attendance. Tension was high, Bini and Felici stood close to the machine while Cerletti and Accornero were watching the patient. The electrodes were placed on the temporal sides of the head, and the machines was set at 80 volts for one tenth of a second. At a nod from the professor,

Bini turned the switch. There was a buzz, and the patient had a sharp contraction, followed by relaxation. . . . In the absence of seizures, however, the treatment was not taking place. Now the question was whether to try again and when to stop before causing harm. The patient had, up to that point, been relatively unconcerned, but when Cerletti ordered that the voltage and duration be increased for another try, he seemed to realize what was happening and said "Careful, the first was pestiferous, the second will be mortiferous" [he had forgotten, according to Accornero, that there had already been two attempts]. Yet even without the seizures, somehow the machine had partly restored his sanity.

Cerletti gave the signal, and a third impulse produced the usual contractions, followed this time by a grand mal seizure. The patient became pale, then cyanotic, and stopped breathing. The corneal reflex disappeared, and tachycardia set in. Accornero was timing the apnea. After 45 seconds there was a big tertorous breath, and then the cyanosis disappeared. (Alverno, 1990: 54–56)

Other versions have the patient awakening "singing a popular song" and "saying something unemotionally about dying" (Kalinowsky, 1982: 3). While Accornero's account describes the attendants as favorable to continuation of the shocks, Impastato (1960: 1113–1114) refers to them as "objecting" to this (quoted in Friedberg, 1976: 134). Unsurprisingly, the more "favorable" descriptions were published in texts favorable to ECT, and vice versa.

Themes associated with twentieth-century EST in Europe and America are reflected in each version of the first electroshock. The patient was lower class and consent was not a paramount issue. From the point of view of the experimenters the patient was "reborn," human communication restored from gibberish, and work roles from uselessness. The patient, however, experienced coma, memory loss, and the fear of death. Follow-up of this first patient (referred to by Endler, 1988a as "S.E."), points to a continuing controversy in the debate over EST: the permanence or impermanence of the changes in behavior or mood that it induces. After 11 shocks, S.E. was "discharged from the Clinic on June 17, 1938, in good condition and well-oriented." But about a year later, although the patient himself (perhaps seeking to avoid shock) said that he was "very well," his wife told a different tale. She reported that "three months after his return home he resumed his jealous attitude toward her and that sometimes during the night he would speak as though in answer to voices" (Endler, 1988a: 16).

ELECTROSHOCK IN THE UNITED STATES

Electroshock came to the United States with European practitioners fleeing fascism and anti-Semitism, an ironic counterpoint to its invention as a tool of fascism. Lothar Kalinowsky, Victor Gonda, Renato Almansi, and others associated with Cerletti migrated to the United States. Almansi fled to the United States in 1939 because of "racial persecution" and brought a

Cerletti machine (Alverno, 1990: 54). Kalinowsky had been working in Cerletti's lab in part to escape the Nazis in his German homeland; later he fled in advance of the German armies to France, Amsterdam, and England before settling permanently in America in March 1940 (Pace, 1992: D23).

It is unclear who performed the "first American EST" but the treatment was instituted in American hospitals by 1940. Perhaps it was the enthusiastic response to EST that prompted a number of independent adaptations of the treatment throughout the United States and thus the many claims to be "the first" (see, for example, Ozarin, 1993 vs. Alverno, 1990). Almansi, together with David Impastato, began using electroshock at Columbus Hospital in New York in February 1940 (Endler, 1988b: 24). Meanwhile, Victor Gonda, a Hungarian neurologist, brought a machine from Europe and began using it on patients in Chicago's Parkway Sanitarium, perhaps in January 1940 (Pulver 1961; Gonda, 1941: 72). Outside of Chicago, Dr. Joseph Zubin of Evanston, Illinois reported to the *Science News Letter* that he was the first American electroshock practitioner (1940). Lothar Kalinowsky, called by historian Edward Shorter the "godparent" of EST in America (1997: 222), is often credited with being the "first." He introduced EST to the New York Psychiatric Institute in September 1940, "where we built a machine of our own" (Endler, 1988a: 21); Kalinowsky remained in practice for the next 50 years, retiring shortly before his death in 1993 (Pace, 1992: D23). Douglas Goldman is yet another candidate for the "first" to use EST in the United States, perhaps because he introduced the psychiatric community to electroshock by demonstrating it in May 1940 at the annual meeting of the American Psychiatric Association in Chicago (Ozarin, 1993: 15; Barton, 1987: 58). Lauren H. Smith, Joseph Hughes, and Donald Hastings were also using electroshock in May of 1940 in Philadelphia, believing that *they* were "the first to start treatment work by this method in this country" (Smith, Hughes, and Hastings, 1941: 452). Alverno (1990: 55) said that American electroshock "was begun almost simultaneously in New York and Chicago at the beginning of 1940, by Victor Gonda and Renato Almansi." Ozarin, in 1993, noted that:

There has been considerable squabbling over who was the first . . . [Barton says] "My investigations show that it was Douglas Goldman in 1939." . . . Barton's excellent account unfortunately fails to quiet the squabbling. His date of 1939 marking Goldman's initial treatment contradicts Goldman's own date of April 1941. (p. 15)

Ozarin concludes that the first American electroshock was given by Impastato on January 7, 1940.

No matter who was first, the professional acceptance of EST can be traced to the 1946 publication of Lothar Kalinowsky and Paul Hoch's *Shock Treatments, Psychosurgery and Other Somatic Treatments*. The treatment was dispersed geographically across the United States from northern and eastern to southern and western hospitals equally pressed by overcrowding and chronic mental illness. Between 1940 and 1943, Delaware, Wisconsin, Massachusetts, New Jersey, Ohio, Illinois, Texas, Louisiana, North Carolina, and South Carolina were among the states adopting EST as a treatment (Philadelphia Psychiatric Society, 1943: 780; Paul, 1942: 86; Cash and Hoekstra, 1941: 851; Myerson, Feldman, and Green, 1941: 1081–1085; Fetterman, 1942: 675; Wanner, 1942: 107; Edlin, 1942: 216–222; Hauser and Barbato, 1941: 228–233; Otis, 1941: 239–242; Lowenbach, 1943: 123–128; Milling, 1943: 182–187). A survey of 305 mental institutions showed that 93 percent of state hospitals had adopted some form of shock therapy by 1935–1941 (Kolb and Vogel, 1942: 92), while in its first two years of use more than 7,000 patients received electric shock in the United States *(Science News Letter,* 1942: 345). A survey of the institutional practices of state hospitals confirms that during the decade between 1940 and 1950 electroshock supplanted other forms of convulsive and somatic therapy. For example, the 1943 *Annual Report of Central State Hospital,* Indianapolis, Indiana, reported that "Electroshock obviates the difficulty of repeated intravenous injections. Patients who have had both forms of therapy prefer electric shock because of its painlessness and because of the lessened malaise" (Central State Hospital, 1943: 19).

Historians have proposed several factors to account for the widespread enthusiasm for electroshock (Berrios, 1997). Electricity, as we have seen, has historically occupied a central place in the cultural imagery of American and European medicine and social life; EST represents a historical continuation of the American fascination with electricity and the machine. Furthermore, the treatment offered a somatic solution in an era of somaticism, while promising greater safety and efficacy than chemically induced convulsions. On a pragmatic level, electroshock required fewer staff to deliver than either Metrazol or insulin. Staff shortages were critical during World War II, which emptied the asylums of personnel. Charles Read, superintendent at Elgin State Hospital in Illinois, noted that his staff dwindled 60 percent during the war, leaving him with 150 openings. He lamented that he had only ten physicians for nearly 5,000 patients (Read, 1945: 275). The shortage of personnel may also explain the decision at East Moline State Hospital in Illinois to discontinue Metrazol after 1942 (East Moline, 1941–1942: 2).

The war also stimulated the search for the diagnosis and treatment of the physical and mental illnesses of combat soldiers; psychiatric casualties were estimated at 500,000 for the army and 150,000 for the navy (Menninger, 1946: 578). When the United States Army turned to Dr. William Menninger to head its psychiatric services, he appointed psychodynamically trained personnel to key military positions. Despite Menninger's professional bias, the electroshock apparatus became part of military medicine.

In 1943 the United States Army, in circular letter no. 88, officially sanctioned electroshock for the treatment of some cases of psychosis (Bernucci and Glass, 1973: 353), and most general hospitals in the Mediterranean theater acquired the equipment (Kavy, 1965: 117–119). The United States Navy equipped hospital ships carrying 75 or more mental patients with EST machines and provided training at psychiatric hospitals at all ports (Menninger, 1948: 321). Despite the fact that distribution of shock machines was uneven—the Southwest Pacific theater had no equipment until 1945 (Bernucci and Glass, 1973: 262)—those physicians who were introduced to electroshock were enthusiastic about the treatment; some hospitals treated upwards of 500 patients with EST (Bernucci and Glass, 1973: 236). For many in the combat zones insulin coma was impractical (Bernucci and Glass, 1973: 82). Overcrowding of mental health facilities was a chronic problem for military personnel (as it was back in the States), and EST seemed to alleviate this. Physicians who tried electroshock found that "The results were remarkable . . . The wild combativeness, the mutism, the hysterical seizures, the paralegias, the aphasia, the deafness, the hyperkinesias, the agitation, the sleeplessness seemed to melt under the effect of electroshock treatment" (Bernucci and Glass, 1973: 148, 149).

TREATMENT BY MACHINE

The vanquishing of other convulsive agents by the electrical machine during the 1940s in America highlights the significance of cultural imagery in medical treatment. As noted in the Introduction, the electrical machine was of considerable significance in the decades of electroshock's introduction and dissemination. Franklin Offner may have been the first to patent a machine in the United States (Barton, 1987: 58–59). Walter Rahm, working at the New York Psychiatric Institute, built an EST machine with the guidance of Lothar Kalinowsky (Kolb, 1993: 70–71). Rahm later worked with Medcraft on its machines (Kolb, 1993: 74). Electrical engineer Reuben Reiter collaborated with psychiatrists Friedman and Wilcox to develop a machine that would deliver EST without the amnesiac problems associated with Bini's device; this machine was to give a greater duration of shock at less amperage (Bromberg, 1982: 125). Taking the opposite tack, in 1945 Douglas Goldman and W.T. Liberson designed a machine that would give a brief shock stimulus (Goldman, 1949: 36–45). Liberson developed a brief-stimulus machine in 1946 that regulated its voltage according to the body's electrical resistance. Unilateral electroshock was developed alongside bilateral, temporal lobe placement alongside anterior-posterior (Friedman, 1942: 218–223). In the 1950s Reiter came out with the Molac II, a reverse glissando treatment that began with an initially high current that was then reduced (Impastato et al., 1957: 381). Over time the equipment became smaller and easier to use (Bale, 1951). Psychiatrists were fascinated with the technology of the machines; in the mid-1950s psychiatrist Milton Greenblatt, then at the Boston Psychopathic Institute, spoke eloquently of "the collaboration of the psychiatrists with the electrical engineer" (Greenblatt, 1955: 93).

In 1948, a group of American psychiatrists listed four main types of machines: the classical alternating-current used by the European experimenters; the controlled-amperage alternating current; the unidirectional pulsating current; and the "Brief stimuli" apparatus (Russell et al., 1948: 74–76). Machines were marketed by Lektra, Medcraft, Offner, Rahm, and Reiter. Psychiatrists in the age of EST, like their electrotherapeutic counterparts, tended to support certain machines and manufacturers. Steinfeld and his colleagues in Pennsylvania mentioned their use of two brand names and models: Offner Machine No. 730 and Medcraft model B24 No. 504. They noted that the Offner model "is set on *calibration* and the time controlled by using a stop watch. We have also employed this machine frequently for glissando shock effects, setting the index on calibration and moving the current control gradually toward a maximum and back" (1951: 144).

The machine occupied the imaginations not only of the psychiatrists who used it, but of the public as well. The EST machine played a prominent role in the 1948 film *The Snake Pit*. When mentally ill protagonist Virginia Cunningham is brought to the EST room she sees the machine; under Antatole Litvak's direction, the camera lingers over the dark and foreboding machine with its large dials. When her psychiatrist pushes the button, dramatic music simulates the convulsion—which is never shown on screen. Indeed, the machine remains on screen for over a minute. The machine also occupies an important role in literature. In "Johnny Panic and the Bible of Dreams," Sylvia Plath described the machine as "A metal box covered with dials and gauges," sitting, snakelike, ready to attack. "The box seems to be eyeing me, copper-head ugly" (Plath, 1968: 60). One EST machine was given an important place in the Eastern Psychiatric booth at the local city-county fair. A sign hung on the machine proudly proclaimed "over 5,000 treatments had been performed" by this single apparatus (Eastern State Hospital, 1999).

Advertisements made the machine the star. In 1940 one of the first advertisements for EST appeared in the *American Journal of Psychiatry*, showing a simple wooden box containing three windows and a dial; the price displayed below the illustration was $275 from Offner Electronics. Subsequent advertisements—which generally showed machines rather than humans—stressed technological improvements. In January 1941 the same machine was advertised with a new description: "New type 730 Apparatus predicts change in a patient's resistance, and precisely determines treatment current" (*American Journal of Psychiatry*, 1941: iii). Rahm Instruments of New York began to compete in the pages of the journal, and it too, showed a small square black box, two windows, and one large dial, all made from solid metal (1942: ii). The power of the marketplace, together with that of the electrical machine, swayed both psychiatrist and patient in mid-twentieth-century America, just as it had in the nineteenth century.

Following World War II, the use of EST increased rapidly: "From the 1940s on, there was hardly a sanitarium, hospital, or private office, that did not use the method" (Bromberg, 1982: 125; see also Moriarty, 1953: 333–338). Some hospitals such as Milledgeville State Hospital in Georgia relied heavily on electroshock, reporting in 1955 that "(5,362) patients were treated and ... (51,321) treatments were given" (Bradford and Peacok, 1955: 24–25). Electroshock spread beyond the confines of state institutions, beyond the disease of schizophrenia and beyond psychiatrists to physicians. Originally targeted at institutionalized patients with chronic psychosis, EST was used by private practice physicians in their office for many neurotic conditions (*Shock for Mental Illness*, 1949: 139; *Fits Produced as Protection*, 1941: 387). The Butler State Hospital *Annual Report* (1953) noted that "Many more psychiatrists are now willing to assume the risk of treating sicker patients in their office practice; electroshock treatment is being administered more liberally on an outpatient basis" (p. 16). In 1946 Polatin reported that EST was indicated in "any type of psychiatric depression of a psychogenic character, such as manic-depressive depressions, senile depressions, involutional depressions, psychoneurotic depressions, and schizophrenic depressions" (p. 174). Some physicians took their machines *out* of the office and made house calls to administer EST (Molle, 1975: 200–221).

As their predecessors had done in the nineteenth century, American EST practitioners formally organized into societies with journals. The Electroshock Research Association began in 1944 (Pallanti, 1999: 630), followed a year later by the Society for Biological Psychiatry (Tourney, 1971: 36). As in the age of electrotherapeutics when the likes of Beard, Rockwell, and Hammond dominated the field, there were "giants" of EST, each with his own "fief." Among the first generation were David Impastato, Lothar Kalinowsky, William Karliner, Sidney Alper, Bernard Pacella, and Frank Gagliardi (Fink, 1994: 67). During the late twentieth century, students and protegés of these men continued to lead the field in research and publication: Max Fink in New York, Harold Sackeim on Long Island, Richard Abrams in Chicago, Charles Kellner in South Carolina, and Richard Weiner in North Carolina.

(HOW) DOES IT WORK?

Throughout the decades since the first American electroshock, researchers have measured its effects in case histories and statistical studies, and attempted to explain the etiology of EST's effect on body, mind, behavior, and symptomatology. As in the previous centuries of medical electricity, electroshock was given to patients with a variety of diagnoses, and at different points in their illness. Last resort, first resort, inpatient, outpatient, prophylactic, and maintenance EST were all mentioned in the research literature during the 1940s–1960s, continuing debates begun in the eighteenth- and nineteenth-century electrotherapeutic literature (see Chapters 1 and 2), and extending into the late twentieth century (see Chapters 4 and 5).

The diagnoses of schizophrenia and psychosis were the first targets of EST treatment, especially in public hospital settings, but the treatment soon spread to less serious diagnoses and to private as well as state hospitals in the United States. In 1951, for example, Steinfeld and his colleagues in Pennsylvania used EST (sometimes in combination with electrical sub-shock, insulin shock, and psychotherapy) for the following diagnoses; schizophrenia, involutional, depressive, manic-depressive, psychoneurotic, paranoic [sic], postpartum, alcoholic, and arteriosclerotic (p. 147). Typically of the pro-EST literature of the time, success rates were reported as high for all diagnoses.

During the 1940s and 1950s, significant post-treatment success rates for electroshock peppered the American clinical literature. In the 1940s, Neyman and his co-workers (1943) concluded that of the 90 schizophrenic patients they treated with ECT, 34.5 percent recovered, with 12.5 percent improved, and 47 percent living outside the hospital. Polatin (1945: 240) reported a 67 to 70 percent "remission" rate for schizophrenics ill for less than six months, which "compares favorably with the spontaneous remission rate of 25 to 30 percent for this same group." Steinfeld and his colleagues, in 1951, noted that most of the 500 EST patients in their sample showed some improvement, measured by shorter (and less expensive) hospital stays (p. 144). However, studies of the longer-term outcome of convulsive treatments were somewhat less optimistic (Neyman et al., 1943: 619; Steinfeld, 1951: 147).

Like their eighteenth- and nineteenth-century predecessors, these electroshock practitioners sought to understand the mechanisms of shock's effect upon body, mind, and behavior. The question for midcentury practitioners was not so much does it work, as how does it work. Both proponents and opponents would probably agree (then and now) that electroshock calms the agitated, and restores the vegetative to interaction. Unlike the nonconvulsive electrical treatments of the nineteenth century and earlier, the effects of EST (since it was the latest in a series of attempted convulsive treatments) were most often presumed to reside in the convulsion, and not in the electricity. From Cerletti onward, researchers who used or observed EST attempted to explain why the convulsions seemed to ameliorate mental symptoms.

Cerletti himself proposed a somatic theory of "vitalizing substances" or "acro-amines" (Valenstein, 1986: 50–51; see also Alverno, 1990: 55), produced in the body in reaction to stress. This theory convinced some French physicians to inject blood from EST patients into the bodies of other schizophrenics (Valenstein, 1986: 52) but without positive results. By 1950 American theories of the operation of EST were legion; one physician cited fifty "popular theories" of why ECT worked (Gordon, 1948: 391–401). In 1945, Polatin noted that because there was no etiological connection between mental disorder and shock, "shock therapies are purely empirical procedures and consequently the exact mechanism is unknown" (p. 288). He summarized the prevailing theories as organic—"major alterations occurring in cerebral metabolism"— and psychological or "psychogenic" (Polatin, 1945: 288).

Some psychiatrists who adopted EST attempted to reconcile the new somatic and apparently successful treatment with older Freudian theories. In their study of EST treatment in a Pennsylvania hospital, Steinfeld and his colleagues linked EST to psychoanalytic theory by arguing that it facilitated transference (1951: 125). They proposed that "To call forth a satisfactory transference from a deeply regressed patient, the therapist often needs to sit with him as he awakens from a shock treatment, judiciously accepting and reciprocating his demonstrations of love" (1951: 129). In his autobiography reflecting on his past experience with electroshock wards, William Sargent commented that "One unit went so far as to recommend nurses with big breasts so that when the patient came out of his death-like coma, he or she was greeted on rebirth with this invitingly maternal sight" (quoted in Porter, 1991: 346).

Psychogenic therapists often saw EST as useful in allowing patients to gain insight into their problems and making them amenable to psychotherapy. Carpenter declared that the "provision of shock fulfills, at least temporarily, a present superego need" (1953: 131). Some patients concurred with these psychoanalytic theories. In 1948 a male electroshock recipient claimed that "Electric shock treatment was successful in my case because there existed a 'love relationship' between myself and Mac [an aide], a relationship such as is established between psychiatrist and patient in narcosynthesis" (Alper, 1948: 207–208). Steinfeld commented on a 34-year-old female "psychoneurotic patient" after a series of four electroshocks: "This treatment-resistant patient wrote . . . 'I wish with all my heart that God and the doctor will help me. . . . I can almost see also the reasons for my 'passion' for the doctor—because he represented so many of the things I have lacked and have been seeking' " (1951: 136).

Mary Jane Ward's popular and semi-autobiographical account of life in a state mental hospital, *The Snake Pit* (1946) married the image of the caring compassionate Freudian doctor Kik with the electric power of the EST machine. The connection between the machine and the cure was heightened in director Anatole Litvak's 1948 film of the book. Virginia Cunningham, played by Olivia de Havilland, is out of touch with reality. Confined to a veritable bedlam of an institution, she meets Dr. Kik, the pipe-smoking, fatherly psychiatrist. The film demonstrates Kik's Freudian emphasis through scenes shot in the doctor's office where a photograph of Sigmund Freud dominates the background. Kik orders EST, and in the following montage we find him charting Virginia's return to reality through electroshock treatment. Once returned to a state of reality she resolves her mental illness through classic Freudian psychoanalysis.

Another set of psychodynamic theories revolved around the association of EST with danger, threat, and punishment. Some physicians suggested that the treatment satisfied the patient's need for punishment. "For example, some patients express eagerness for the treatment; there is a masochistic element behind the desire for treatment" (Millet and Mosse, 1944: 352). One psychodynamic theory was that the seizure released a patient's pent-up aggression and hostility through the violent muscular convulsions. Perhaps the patient experienced shock as a threat to her life, against which she mobilized. Or, perhaps the apparent danger of the procedure made the patient's family treat her better after it (Alexander and Selesnick, 1966: 283–284). These ideas were incorporated into the treatment techniques of a growing number of psychodynamic psychiatrists, but were also used against EST by other members of the psychiatric community—a group that would become more vocal as the century progressed (see Chapters 4 and 5).

Physiological theories about the operation of electroshock were just as numerous and speculative as the psychodynamic. Some researchers suggested that electroshock stimulated the hypothalamus and affected the sympathetic nervous system. Another theory was that the brain got caught in a sort of feedback loop that needed to be reversed by EST (Alexander and Selesnick, 1966: 283–284). Despite their psychoanalytic orientation and transference mechanism theory of EST, the Pennsylvania researchers also theorized that EST worked by changing the chemistry of the blood and creating acidosis (Steinfeld, 1951: 221–223).

Some psychosomatic theories focused on the immediate postconvulsive effects of EST, since all patients seemed to have memory difficulties and some displayed aphasia (Shryock, 1947: 61). Steinfeld and his colleagues noted that "an organically induced amnesia serves as a 'breathing spell' to the patient from the present onslaught of his id impulses, and enables him to establish a transference" (1951: 122). Other physicians proposed that the post-EST "marked organic confusion and memory defect" might "in themselves comprise the therapeutically beneficial elements of the treatment" (Alexander, 1953: 61). It was this line of thought that prompted Bini to advocate what he called "annihilation therapy," or multiple, repeated, daily dosages of shock on psychotic patients (Cerletti, 1950: 94). One patient received 1,000 treatments in a period of ten years with no reported side effects (Polatin and Philtine, 1949: 149).

Researchers devised experiments to try to determine whether electroshock worked organically or psychodynamically. In a study comparing insulin or Metrazol shock with electricity, Neyman and his colleagues (1943: 624) first told their patients that they were being taken into a room for the purpose of studying their brain waves. They did this to control the "fear effect." The researchers said that "Later these precautions of deliberately misleading the patients were dropped. We became convinced that in most cases emotions and especially fear played little if any part in the success or failure of the treatment" (1943: 624). It became clear that the means by which EST cured would remain unknown. No theories could be proven, and the "curative" mechanism "remains obscure" (Aldrich, 1955: 176). One textbook noted that "The rationale, other than that based on its empirical value . . . still is to a large extent obscure" (Alexander, 1953: 60).

Practitioners throughout the century debated the machinery, amperage, voltage, and calibration of EST, and the ideal duration and number of treatments. In general, the twentieth-century trend has been from "less" to "more" in the complexity and calibration of machines; from "more" to "less" in electroshock's administration. Although electrical treatment has been presented to the public as a treatment of "last resort," practitioners since the eighteenth century have proposed it as a treatment of first resort. As in the eighteenth and nineteenth centuries, pushbutton psychiatry appeared in both the asylum and the outpatient clinic. And, while there have been arguments throughout the decades for the limitation of the treatment to particular diagnoses, the general trend has been to expand the mental illness and even physical illness diagnoses for which it is used, as in its recent use in Parkinson's disease. However, what has remained constant is the gender hierarchy within which these changing techniques are practiced. As in the nineteenth century, those mainstream physicians who practiced electrical psychiatry were male (Frankel et al., 1978: 5), while the majority of their patients, by the 1950s, were female (Warren, 1987: 25).

PATIENTS AT MIDCENTURY: MADWIVES IN *THE BELL JAR*

In the case histories of electroshock practitioners we find reported the incidences, diagnoses, successes and failures of the procedure; accounts which can be used to assess the association between the treatment and hierarchies of gender, class, race/ethnicity, and age. Prevalent in the United States during the 1950s, EST was available at both public and private hospitals with few insurance barriers, making it available to all social classes and all age groups, including children (Bender, 1947) and the elderly (Feldman et al., 1946: 158–170). Although there were minority recipients of ECT, this new form of electrical treatment was associated with the Anglo, Caucasian patient, as many nineteenth-century electrical treatments had been (Fink, 1994b: 242). But the most consistent and lasting association with EST was with gender.

The association between EST and gender was quantitative, but it was also what Showalter and others call metaphorical, reflecting (with its associated diagnoses of hysteria and neurasthenia), the place of women in Western society. Some of the early statistical studies of EST, however, reported roughly as many men as women shock recipients—45 and 47, respectively, for example, in Neyman et al.'s 1943 study. Other studies did not count by gender. Steinfeld and his colleagues, for example, reported on a sample of 500 patients drawn randomly from 900 EST recipients at a Pennsylvania Hospital. None of their tables used gender as a variable, although it is clear that the 17 postpartum diagnoses were of women patients (1951: 147). Their illustrative case histories, however, were almost all of women patients: in one chapter, the histories of 21 women and 1 man were given.

Electroshock was, as are perhaps all psychiatric treatments, deeply implicated in the gender and family role relations of the world of 1950s America. This era is legendary for its invocation of traditional gender roles, with the woman responsible for the internal and domestic (May, 1988), and the man for the external and public, arenas of social life (Goffman, 1961)—and for sexuality (Warren, 1987). Neyman and his American colleagues, like Aldini in Italy a century and a half earlier, "judged a patient recovered if on reexamination he showed no psychotic symptoms, if his family considered him well, and if he was able to resume the same or a higher status in the community" (1943: 631–632). This patient appears to be literally, as well as linguistically, a "he." Rickles and Olson (1948: 339) noted that a female patient was considered well if she could "manage her home efficiently" or become "active in society."

Electroshock occupied an ironic space between electrical household machinery and psychiatric treatment by electric machine. From 1917 to 1940 the number of American households electrified rose from less than 25 percent to more than 90 percent, and American consumption was not, overall, affected by the Depression (Chant, 1989: 102). The middle class of the 1940s was devoted to electrically powered machines for household operation: vacuum cleaners, washers, dryers, irons, toasters, and electric stoves were marketed to the American woman as "efficient" and "modern." These machines did not release her from the domestic sphere but, rather, confined her ever more closely (Chant, 1989: 102; Adas, 1980: 409). One journalist, introduced to EST by Lothar Kalinowsky at the New York Psychiatric Institute, imagined a patient "cured simply in his own home by a physician," who after putting the electrodes in place "just plugs into an ordinary household current" (Van De Water, 1940: 42). Indeed, EST machines in their own way—much as other domestic appliances—sought to make a woman more efficient in her home, and any protestations about a woman's traditional role might be silenced at the push of a button on an EST machine. As one journalist noted:

Take the case of the middle-aged woman who had been a civic leader in her community until she became a victim of mental depressions that virtually confined her to her home. She gave up her outside interests and became careless in her personal appearance, spent a great deal of time in weeping, and required constant supervision. Following six electric shock treatments, this woman was able to resume her normal way of life. She was not only able to manage her household as before and return to her clubs and her civic organizations, but she took on the added task of hunting out other persons she thought might be benefited by electric shock treatment. (Shryock 1947: 60)

Not all mad housewives were as sanguine about electroshock as this woman, although many husbands and mothers-in-law liked the effect it had on their wives and daughters-in-law (Warren, 1987).

As in Victorian and ancient times, women in mid-twentieth-century America were liable to be seen as mentally disordered in the context of their reproductive functions (menstruation, childbirth, menopause), as well as their gender role "duties" as wives and mothers. Describing a married female patient who exhibited "marked improvement" after EST, Steinfeld and his colleagues commented that "the patient, for the first time since her marriage, accepted her husband completely and did not reject his desire for impregnating her" (1951: 186). A marriage manual published in 1952 warned that a woman's menstrual cycle and her attendant mood changes could "harm her marriage greatly if she does not handle this intelligently" (Popenoe, 1952: 124). If she did not control her mood swings she was to consider "Administration of hormones . . . in more serious instances electric shock may produce satisfactory results" (Popenoe, 1952: 124).

Madwives, women who defied their social role, faced the joint power of marital and psychiatric expertise. "Mr. N," a husband quoted in Popenoe's manual, said, "You bet I watch the calendar. . . . It would help a lot in our home if she would learn how to handle herself at that time of the month instead of just giving way to her feelings" (1952: 124). The husbands in the Bay Area study of 17 diagnosed schizophrenic women and their families (Sampson, Messinger, and Towne, 1969; Warren, 1987) monitored their wives' domestic behavior for signs of mental instability. Symptoms included not doing the housework adequately or (conversely) overdoing housework, and a desire to work outside the home. Out-of-line ambitions, appearances, behavior, or sexuality were symptomatized; hospitalization and EST were proposed to restore 1950s madwives to their social place as well as to their senses. The themes of thwarted ambition (and at times sexuality) and the self's suffocation within traditional gender roles appeared in women's writings of the mid-twentieth century.

The literary representation of electroshock at midcentury is darkly gendered, reflecting the ancient association of electricity with the polarities of death-rebirth and dominance-submission. Virginia, the protagonist in *The Snake Pit*, experienced EST as electrocution, being punished and killed without a trial (Ward, 1946: 43), as did Sylvia Plath, whose character wondered "what terrible thing it was I had done" (1971: 116–117). In her autobiographical novel *The Bell Jar*, Plath described her "return from the dead" through EST (1971: 175). For Plath, the treatment fused the images of electroshock, wedlock, death, and rebirth: "Something old, something new . . . but I wasn't getting married. There ought, I think, to be a ritual for being born twice" (1971: 199). The EST procedure evoked sexuality for Plath as well, reminding her of her father's "penis dangling behind a loosely tied bathrobe . . . the charisma of my father's assertive mind and temperament" (1972: 21).

The gender and sexual imagery of EST in *The Bell Jar* is reminiscent of the genital electrotherapeutics of the eighteenth and nineteenth centuries, and their origins in Galen's widow's treatment (see the Preface). The joining of the electrical and the genital in the treatment of mental disorder that we saw from the mideighteenth to early twentieth century had all but disappeared from electroshock, with its focus on the brain. But menstruation was still linked by some mid-twentieth-century psychiatrists to mental illness, as it had been for more than two thousand years (see the Preface). Steinfeld and his colleagues, for example, gave monthly shock treatments to 27 percent of all their female patients, and 40 percent of all their postpartum patients, saying that "monthly treatments for female patients have special significance . . . the menstrual period, especially shortly after a patient's discharge from the hospital is critical and certain types more prone to the effects of menstrual depression are given shock treatments at about these times at monthly intervals" (1951: 148).

These researchers also treated some of their female patients with male hormones, alone or with EST. The logic of the hormone treatment was to break down sexual inhibitions by encouraging "direct genital gratification," accomplished by increasing clitoral excitability. The resulting genital pleasure, as in the case of Galen's widow, would then provide "alleviation . . . of some of the symptoms" of mental disorder through masturbation" (1951: 207–208). The Pennsylvania physicians noted that "We administered testosterone propionate to . . . 'frigid' psychotic patients to increase the clitoris excitability and thus the urge for sexual gratification. Altogether nine patients were treated with this aim in mind. All of them responded with a heightened sexual excitability and some improvement in their capacity for adjustment" (1951: 209). In the case of a female "psychoneurotic," aged 22, treated with 24 sub-coma insulin treatments with 14 superimposed electroshocks: "The therapist . . . spent considerable time with the patient. . . . She began to form a strong positive transference, the very intensity and *genital character* of which was later to clash with her weakened, aggressive ego" (1951: 138; italics added). Females who did not have a heterosexual orientation or who had "unacceptable homosexual trends" were also subject to electroshock (Gronner, 1945: 64).

Although roughly two thirds of mid-century electroshock patients were women, men were also hospitalized and given ECT in the context of gender and sexual roles. Males who deviated from the prescribed sexual interest in females became liable for EST and other treatments. A 23-year-old African American man was hospitalized for homosexual behavior and disturbing the peace. Given eight electroshocks between December 19, 1941 and January 5, 1942, his doctor noted "With electroshock therapy, the patient recovered from his psychosis and his transvestism although he remained overtly homosexual" (quoted in Katz, 1976: 173; see also Adair and Adair, 1978). When his lifestyle and homosexuality became an issue Lou Reed was given electro-shock to "cure" him (Bockris, 1994).

Male EST patients in the 1950s and 1960s who behaved in ways unbecoming to men of their times were subject to treatment. Leonard Frank, diagnosed as a "severe and chronic" "paranoid schizophrenic," and treated through-out the 1960s with drugs, insulin coma, and EST, was seen as in rebellion against parental and religious authority. The "Frank papers" document the centrality of his beard as a symbol of revolt. To Frank his beard was symbolic of the religious orthodoxy he cherished; to his father and his psychiatrist, it was a symbol of defiance: "Well into the shock series . . . the treating psychiatrist wrote to my father . . . 'he still has all his delusional beliefs regarding his beard, dietary regime, and religious observances that he had prior to treat-ment.' During the comatose phase of one of my treatments, my beard was removed—as a 'therapeutic device to provoke anxiety and make some change in his body image' " (Frank, 1990: 490).

But, like women's domestic work, men's work outside the home was of crucial significance in the process of mental illness diagnosis, treatment, and outcome assessment during the 1940s–1960s for both family members and physicians. His wife said of "Robert," a 35-year-old cab driver hospitalized with a diagnosis of schizophrenia, that he chased her around the house while growling like a lion, and lost interest in work. "For a cab driver he worked hard. . . . When he felt good. . . . He didn't work so hard when he didn't" (Yarrow, Schwartz, and Deasy, 1955; see also Warren, 1983). Among Steinfeld's case histories was a man, T.E., diagnosed as involutional. Inter-twined among descriptions of his hallucinations and delusions are com-ments on his working or not working: "He had seemed to adjust himself fairly well [after EST] and had worked satisfactorily at three temporary jobs. Two weeks before his readmission he had again become depressed, restless, and had auditory hallucinations . . . and was unable to continue with his work" (1951: 172–173).

Just as electroshock triumphed in American psychiatry, opinions about the treatment began to undergo a radical change, and it was during the late 1950s that the stage was set for psychiatric, legal, lay, and patient challenges to the treatment. The electrical and technical enthusiasm for pushbutton psychiatry, with its emphasis on conformity, normality, and fixed gender roles, and the almost unified psychiatric embrace of EST, would be eroded by a new era of social tumult, rejection of technology, and the joined potency of media and patients' voices.

Chapter 4

Rage Against the Machine: The Decline of Electroshock, 1966–1980

At the push of a button by the physician when all is in readiness, the patient instantaneously becomes unconscious, undergoes convulsions and lapses into what resembles a profound sleep. Upon awakening from the coma, many shout loudly as if in pain, though no pain is experienced. The female patients who are more communicative about their feelings tend to exaggerate this distaste—a female said, characteristically "I don't know whether they have their degrees or not but I don't want to be submitted to anymore of these treatments. They line you up regularly; it is a hard and fast rule to take the treatments—Are there no human rights at all?"
—H. Warren Dunham and S. Kirkson Weinberg, 1960

The American political and social upheavals of the late 1960s and early 1970s gave rise to an era of patients' civil rights, prompted the "decarceration" or "deinstitutionalization" of the asylum, challenged professional assumptions about what it meant to be mad—and drove electroshock, for a time, into the borderland of psychiatric practice. The ideologies of individual rights, collective identity, and social freedom formed the background to the emergence of the anti-psychiatry and anti-ECT movements in the 1970s. These movements were led by ex-patients, social scientists, lawyers, and anti-ECT psychiatrists, and were widely publicized in the media. Like its predecessor, the nineteenth-century Alleged Lunatics Friends Society (Sapinsky, 1991: xii), the twentieth-century patients' rights movement opposed involuntary confinement in institutions in addition to involuntary ECT, and in some cases voluntary ECT.

During the 1960s the concept of mental illness itself, and the legitimacy of psychiatry as a medical specialty, came under the scrutiny of scholars in Europe and America. Mental illness was reframed as labeling, and psychiatry as social control. French intellectual Michel Foucault (1973) suggested that insanity was a cultural construct invented in the eighteenth century; the asylum functioned to control the behavior of the unreasonable in the age of reason. On the other side of the channel, British psychiatrist R.D. Laing proposed that schizophrenia was not a disease but, rather, a strategy of coping with destructive circumstances (Laing, 1969: 102–103).

These reframings of insanity and its cures were echoed in the United States. Sociologist Erving Goffman (1961) portrayed asylums as sites of social control, and the symptomatic behavior of patients as self-protective strategies. Both Goffman and fellow-sociologist Thomas Scheff (1966) pointed to the use of everyday-life norm violations as an aspect of psychiatric diagnosis. Howard Becker (1961) proposed the labeling theory of deviance, in which madness is constituted by the reactions to it (from observation to psychiatric labeling) rather than anything intrinsic to it. Even psychiatry had its labeling theorist: Thomas Szasz (1961) wrote of psychiatry as parallel to witchcraft. These ideas, particularly those of Foucault and Goffman, were influential in an interdisciplinary scholarship of social control that flourished in America from the 1970s onward (see, for example, Rothman 1971; Grob, 1977; Staples, 1991). These intellectual currents joined with the popular media in portraying electroshock in *One Flew Over the Cuckoo's Nest*.

The most powerful imagery of electroshock from this era was the book (Kesey, 1962) and film (1975) *One Flew Over the Cuckoo's Nest*; this work placed EST at the center of the anti-machine, anti-technology critique of the time. In this popular anti-establishment work, electroshock appeared as part of the mechanized, machine-centered, emotionless world. *Cuckoo's Nest* exemplified scholarly and popular images of the mental institution as a site of repression, electroshock as punishment, and society as constructing mental illness and applying disease labels to social deviants. Indeed, protagonist Randall McMurphy is portrayed as troubled and deviant but not mentally ill. But because of his refusal to accept social authority, he is forced to undergo a series of increasingly drastic treatment/punishments, culminating in EST and, finally, lobotomy and physical, as well as social death.

Patients in the novel are described as "machines with flaws inside" who were taken to the shock shop for "repair" (Kesey, 1962: 19), a metaphor echoed in the words of actual patients: "My own head was used for a wall socket," said one, "it was as if I was being murdered many times" (Moran, 1952: 146). The novel's action takes place in the ward of "Big Nurse," who fights McMurphy for control of the ward. Nurse Ratched is the embodiment of an emotionless social engineer. She carries around a bag shaped like a tool box "full of a thousand parts . . . wheels and gears, cogs polished to a hard glitter, tiny pills that gleam like porcelain, needles, forceps, watchmaker's pliers, rolls of copper wire" (Kesey, 1962: 19). McMurphy, representing those who resist social or gender conventions, is introduced to the "shock shop" and ECT—"A device that might be said to do the work of the sleeping pill, the electric chair, and the torture rack"—learning that the ECT machine is as modern as any kitchen appliance: "It's a clever little procedure, simple, quick, nearly painless, it happens so fast" (Kesey, 1962, 64). "You are strapped to a table, shaped, ironically, like a cross, with a crown of electric spikes in place of thorns," then "Five cents worth of electricity through the brain and you are jointly administered therapy and punishment for your hostile go-to-hell behavior" (Kesey, 1962: 64–65).

But it was not only culture and its images that banished electroshock, for a brief interlude, to the hinterland. Important structural, legal, and economic changes relevant to ECT occurred in American society during the late 1960s and early 1970s, including the deinstitutionalization and patients' rights movements, the development of "newer and better" psychopharmacology, and changes in the ways in which hospitals and doctors were organized and financed. Those Freudian and other anti-ECT psychiatrists who had remained opposed to electroshock even during its heyday found themselves in a position to take their case, once more, to the mainstream of American psychiatry.

ELECTROSHOCK AND ORGANIZED PSYCHIATRY

Electroshock had been used throughout the 1940s and 1950s by psychiatrists and even Freudian analysts who saw in it a useful tool for preparing patients for psychotherapy and analysis (see Chapter 3). However, within the analytical community there had always been psychiatrists who opposed somatic treatments and adhered to a strict Freudian approach, claiming that mental illness was caused by mental rather than physical problems. These psychodynamic psychiatrists, or "psychikers," opposed somatically inclined psychiatrists, or "somatikers," who sought a physical etiology of mental illness. Working through institutions such as the Menninger Foundation and professional affiliations such as the Group for the Advancement of Psychiatry (GAP), psychikers for a time dominated the American Psychiatric Association (APA), even as electroshock treatment spread throughout the country. Individuals supportive of a psychodynamic theory of mental illness, such as the Menninger brothers Karl and William, wielded considerable social and political influence both within the profession of psychiatry and among the general public. In 1946, William C. Menninger and 13 colleagues founded the GAP, which challenged the APA to "modernize" (Grob, 1991: 191–198). Some GAP members held positions within the APA from which they emphasized psychodynamic theories and therapies (Grob, 1991: 197–199). At the same time, Karl Menninger chaired a special committee established to reorganize the APA (Grob, 1991: 25).

Karl and William also worked from their base at the Menninger Clinic in Topeka, Kansas, to develop strong ties with the government. Dr. William Menninger's experience with the military no doubt assisted in the award of a contract from the government in the late 1940s to develop a psychiatric residency program at a former VA hospital in Topeka. Opened in 1946, the Menninger School of Psychiatry (MSP) trained half of all VA psychiatrists and over a third of all psychiatric residents in the United States. In the immediate postwar years this training accounted for 15 percent of American psychiatrists (Friedman, 1990: 179, 199). The hospital also became the site for a doctoral program in clinical psychologists sponsored by the University of Kansas and the Veterans Administration (VA) and funded through the National Institutes of Mental Health (NIMH) and thus the Menningers and their associates influenced the postwar development of clinical psychology as well as psychiatry (Grob, 1991: 51).

GAP members were often anti-ECT. Robert Knight, who had worked at the Menninger Foundation, attacked what he called "strong arm" therapies, including shock (Grob, 1991: 37). In 1947 the GAP Committee on Therapy, chaired by M. Ralph Kauffman, initiated an attack on ECT in its first report on the state of psychiatry. GAP's Committee on Therapy noted ECT's "promiscuous and indiscriminate" use, and cited the following problems: 1) no theory of its mode of action; 2) conflicting evidence of its efficacy in the schizophrenias; 3) contra-indications with psychoneuroses; and 4) complications and hazards. "Widespread abuses" of electroshock included its use in office rather than hospital practice and its use with too many diagnoses and as the sole therapeutic agent (Blain papers, 1948: box 9). Although William Menninger himself had conceded that ECT might be applicable in five or ten percent of all psychiatric cases (Freeman, 1956: 255), the GAP report led the Los Angeles Medical Society to expel members who used ECT in their offices (Pressman, 1998: 378).

To some extent problems cited in the GAP report were recognized by ECT practitioners. From the beginning even enthusiastic practitioners had visceral reactions to the treatment, including Cerletti (see Frank, 1990: 493; Porter, 1991: 334) and Kalinowsky. Cerletti's initial report indicated that patients had clonic jerks and spasms, their faces turned from red to white to blue, and then the patient "foams at the mouth, ejaculates, or passes urine" (Cerletti, 1938: 260). After witnessing his first electroshock, Kalinowsky reportedly told his wife, "I saw something terrible today—I never want to see that again" (Frank, 1990: 492). Zigmond Lebensohn, another early electroshock pioneer, recalled, "The first time I witnessed electroconvulsive treatment in 1939, I had some of the same visceral reaction I experienced as a medical student witnessing my first medical operation" (1984: 39). One psychiatrist cautioned that "All this [ECT] may sound very terrifying to the physician who is not intimately acquainted with electric shock therapy" (Neyman et al., 1943: 619).

Indeed, for physicians unacquainted with ECT the practice raised a number of questions about the safety and efficacy of the treatment. During the 1940s, psychiatrists used a potentially dangerous combination of drugs to prevent the broken bones and fractures associated with the early use of electroshock. Patients received curare before the treatment to relax their muscles, then strychnine afterward to restart their breathing ("Depression and Electroshock," *Newsweek*, 7 August 1972: 20). Kalinowsky called ECT "the most abused treatment in modern psychiatry" and thought that over-use would continue because of the "greater efficiency in the manufacture of the instruments" and their "compactness" that put the equipment in the hands of individuals with little training (Kalinowsky, 1948: 161, 170). How-ever, when threatened by the GAP report, the somatikers counterattacked.

GAP reconsidered its first report in the face of somatiker pressure. William Menninger attempted to pacify the somatikers by writing to Theodore Robie that it was the unprofessional practice of ECT that was at fault, not necessarily ECT itself. "I think I related to you that an acquaintance of mine," wrote Menninger, "one of our former members of the Army, who has never had any psychiatric training, gives to my knowledge from ten to twenty-five shocks a day in his office in a large city in Iowa" (Blain papers, 1948: box 9). GAP created a revised Committee on Therapy and invited the principal proponents of ECT, including Kalinowsky and Paul Hoch, to sit in on the committee as consultants, even allowing the "self-appointed defender of electroshock," Theodore Robie, to speak as a guest (Blain papers, 1948: box 9). The revised GAP report published August 1, 1950 eliminated criticism of the office use of ECT.

Psychiatric criticism of shock also focused on the issue of what the treatment might do to the brain, nervous system, or body of the patient. Neurologists and clinical psychologists had, from the 1940s onward, speculated on and investigated the physical effects of electroshock (Fleishinger, 1945: 185; Ebaugh, 1943: 107; Gralnick, 1945: 189). Whereas the electroshock propo-nents denied evidence of brain damage (Barrera et al., 1942: 31–35), neurology and psychology texts pointed to possible "side effects" such as brain damage (Baker, 1955: 1029; Janis, 1950a: 359–382; 1950b: 383–397), or brain hemorrhage (Alpers and Hughes, 1942a: 173; 1942b: 385). Professional discussions of the effects of EST came to public attention when *Science News Letter* published an article charging that "Electric Shock Causes Partial Memory Loss" (1940: 182).

These various critiques of ECT received greater attention in the late 1960s and 1970s when anti-ECT psychiatrists joined ex-patients in the media and legislative fights against ECT. During the 1970s, neurologist John Friedberg published *Shock Treatment Is Not Good for Your Brain* (1976), while psychiatrist Peter Breggin founded the anti-ECT Center for the Study of Psychiatry and wrote extensively on the brain- and memory-damaging ef-fects of ECT (Breggin, 1991). At the 129th annual meeting of the APA in Mi-ami Beach in 1976, Friedberg claimed that "From a neurological point of view ECT is a method of producing amnesia by selectively damaging the temporal and the structures within them. ECT produces a form of brain disease" (Friedberg, 1977: 100). Friedberg quoted psychiatrist Paul Hoch, who co-authored an important ECT text with Lothar Kalinowsky, as asking if "a certain amount of brain damage [is] not necessary for this type of treat-ment?" (1976: 139).

The writings of anti-ECT experts were filtered to the general public through the mass media during the 1970s and early 1980s. Fueling public interest in electroshock in the early 1970s was Senator Thomas Eagleton's decision to withdraw as a vice-presidential candidate in the 1972 presidential election. Eagleton's decision came after revelations that between 1960 and 1972 he had been hospitalized for depression three times and that his treatment included EST ("Problem a Closed Chapter," *Chicago Tribune*, 26 July 1972: 4). At issue for the public was the mental stability of Eagleton; it could not have helped him to have a spokesman for the American Psychological Association claim that electroshock was "more of a last-resort treatment for the severely depressed and potentially suicidal" ("Shock Therapy: What it Means," *Chicago Tribune*, 26 July 1972: 4). The public perception of EST can be detected in the response to a 1975 article in *Psychology Today* by Friedberg, "Electroshock Therapy: Let's Stop Blasting the Brain." The publication received some 50 responses to this article, 32 supporting the article's anti-EST stance (Friedberg, 1975: 10). Friedberg claimed to have received another 58 letters opposed to EST, 38 from "victims" (Friedberg, 1975: 10). The public's antipathy toward EST was also indicated in a survey of media depictions of EST by Kalayam and Steinhart (1981). They found that while some depictions were positive and some balanced in their depiction of ECT, many "depicted ECT as an inhuman and sadistic form of treatment administered by doctors and nurses" (p. 185).

The response of the proponents of electroshock within the APA to the various media and public critiques was to pressure their organization to engage in a thorough investigation of the clinical literature on shock. In 1978 the APA, according to one ECT proponent, "issued a full and careful analysis of the place of ECT in medical/psychiatric practice" (Greenblatt, 1984: 1409). This report was, in Greenblatt's words, based on "the considerable further advance in technology and clinical experience" with ECT since 1940 (1984b: 1409). A survey of members' attitudes in 1978 led the APA to conclude that 67 percent of the members were favorable to ECT, 32 percent somewhat unfavorable, and only 2 percent completely opposed (Greenblatt 1984b: 1409).

But anti-ECT sentiment was not the only source of challenge to electroshock treatment within the profession. Earlier developments in pharmacology had also, by the 1960s and 1970s, set the stage for somatic alternatives to ECT. Although drug treatment is as ancient as the madness it treats, the drugs developed since the 1950s in America had been heralded as both liberating and revolutionary. Antidepressants such as amitriptyline and elavil were developed during the 1950s (Barton 1987: 226), while chlorpromazine (CPZ), a treatment for severe mental illness, was introduced in 1954 by Smith, Kline, and French of Philadelphia under the name Thorazine (Swazey, 1974: 159). Both psychotherapists and ECT practitioners initially resisted the new drug treatments (Swazey, 1974: 202); in response,

Smith, Kline, and French expanded its sales force and government and hospital lobbying activities (Shorter, 1987: 124). Eight months after its introduction in 1954, CPZ was being prescribed to more than two million patients (Keisler and Sibulkin, 1987). The use of psychopharmacology prompted a decrease in ECT use in some places during the late 1950s: Veterans Administration (VA) hospitals in one year alone (1955–1956) decreased the number of ECT treatments by 25 percent (Swazey, 1974: 219). In a study of Elgin State Hospital, the author found that "electroshock had almost completely ceased by 1961, as antidepressant drugs were found to be more effective" (Briska, 1971: 43).

The drug industry took ECT to task directly, advertising in the *Diseases of the Nervous System* (August 1955) that "Thorazine reduces the need for electroshock therapy." Included in the advertisement was a testimonial from a physician at Rochester State Hospital that "most of the electric shock in the hospital was suddenly abolished" and replaced by Thorazine. A similar item appeared in the *American Journal of Psychiatry*, where the first page of a two-page advertisement showed a bespectacled male physician wearing a white lab coat. The physician had one hand on the ECT machine and the other clamping a male patient's mouth shut. The second page proclaimed, "ECT replaced in 57 percent of depressed patients with Deprol" (1958: xii). The impact of pharmacology on the profession is demonstrated by the fact that psychiatrists trained in the United States between 1965 and 1985 did not consider ECT "a needed skill" (Fink & Bailine, 1998: 108).

PATIENTS' VOICES AGAINST ELECTROSHOCK

ECT came under attack, during the 1970s, not only from psychiatrists, pharmacologists, scholars, and the mass media, but also by patients. The late 1960s and early 1970s were a time of tumultuous social change, political activism, and cultural critique: a cusp between the modern and the postmodern eras in America. The civil rights movement sought to extend human freedoms to still-disenfranchised African Americans, while the latest wave of the feminist movement drew attention to the second-class place of women both in society as a whole and, ironically, within the civil rights movement. The gay liberation movement began in earnest, as did the era's critique of war, environmental pollution, and technology. In contrast to the 1890s, 1930s, and 1950s fascination with the machine, fear of the machine informed the literature and social science of the times (Roszak, 1969; Reich, 1970). The patients' rights and anti-ECT movement emerged from this crucible of social change.

The patients' rights movement gave voice to patients both individually and collectively. In December 1973, Leonard Frank and another ex-patient, Wade Hudson, founded the Network Against Psychiatric Assault (NAPA). Ted Chabinski, who received shock as a child under the care of Dr. Lauretta

Bender, formed another patients' advocacy group and published the *Madness Network News*. Continuing his struggle against ECT through the 1980s, Chabinski formed the Coalition to Stop Electroshock and engineered a 1982 referendum banning ECT in Berkeley, California (Isaac and Armat, 1990: 206). Marilyn Rice, a bureaucrat with the Department of Commerce in the 1960s, described her memory (and employment) loss in NAPA's "Shock Packet" (1975). Later in 1984 Rice founded the Committee for Truth in Psychiatry (CTIP) (Cameron, 1994: 179) to encourage the FDA to regulate ECT machines; when Rice died in 1992, Linda Andre became director of CTIP.

The focus of anti-shock activism in the decades of the 1970s and 1980s centered on the issues of ECT destroying important aspects of patients' personalities and memories, and forcible shock violating their civil rights. Ernest Hemingway is said to have lamented to visiting A.E. Hochner at the Mayo Clinic in 1961: "Well, what is the sense of ruining my head and erasing my memory, which is my capital, and putting me out of business? It was a brilliant cure, but we lost the patient" (Frank, 1990: 508). Patients as diverse as the hippie Mark Vonnegut (1975), the religious Leonard Frank (1990), and the bureaucrat Marilyn Rice (1974) also spoke of the erasure of self through ECT. In 1990, Frank recalled that his earlier treatment "destroyed large parts of my memory, including the two-year period preceding the last shock" (p. 490). Marilyn Rice commented on her shock-induced loss of memory, "The work in which I was engaged was specifically dependent upon the fund of knowledge I had determinedly accumulated over more than twenty years." When she sought further treatment to cope with unexpected memory loss, her physician, echoing the intersection of gender roles with psychiatry characteristic of the 1950s, told her "your work was too big a part of your life" (Frank, 1978: 92–99).

Mark Vonnegut, son of the novelist Kurt Vonnegut, was diagnosed as schizophrenic and involuntarily hospitalized during the same era as Frank's beard dispute. Although he finally decided that he was mentally ill and needed hospitalization, Vonnegut invoked the labeling theory of deviance current in scholarship and hippie culture alike, and its paradoxical relation to serious mental symptomatology:

What could they [his friends] do? Putting someone in a nut house isn't a nice thing to do to someone. There are lots of pressures in the hip community that make that sort of decision even harder to come to than normally. Doctors don't know anything, mental hospitals are repressive, fascist, etc. "Schizophrenia is a sane response to an insane society. . . . Mental illness is a myth." (Vonnegut, 1975: 143)

Demonstrations by NAPA and other groups sought to interest laypeople and politicians in the plight of ECT ex-patients by targeting hospitals that used ECT, especially in California (Frank, 1978: 109). A monthly radio program on WBAI-FM in New York City broadcast the complaints of the ex-patients to the public (Dain, 1989: 10). The media, perhaps influenced by the popularity of *Cuckoo's Nest,* raised questions as to the role of psychiatry in general. In May 1977, one network ran promotions for an upcoming television documentary on *Madness and Medicine* stating that "Doctors drug them, shock them, cut into their brains, but do they do any good?," prompting the APA to complain to the Federal Communications Commission (FCC) citing the Fairness Doctrine (Frankel, 1982: 246).

Additional attacks on psychiatry came from L. Ron Hubbard, the science-fiction writer who launched the Church of Scientology in the mid-1950s. Hubbard, whose doctrine was that behavioral changes occurred through mechanical reprogramming of brain "engrams," claimed that ECT created dangerous engrams in the brain (Shorter, 1997: 282); clearly, shock machinery was in competition with Scientology's own engram-changing machines. The Church of Scientology created the Citizen's Commission on Human Rights (CCHR), and initially hired Thomas Szasz as its consulting psychiatrist (Shorter, 1997: 283). The CCHR successfully challenged ECT in Texas, which led to legislative oversight and some of the toughest laws regulating the use of ECT anywhere in the nation (see below).

Although a feminist critique of ECT was nascent in the writings of 1950s patients such as Sylvia Plath, by the early 1970s it had crystallized into a new intellectual and social movement. Feminists and female ex-patients of this era noted that women were predominantly the recipients of ECT, receiving 70.1 percent of ECT treatments for affective disorder nationwide in 1975 and 64.5 percent in 1980 (Thompson and Blaine, 1987: 559); Morrisey, Steadman, and Burton (1981) comment that for 1972–1977 in New York, "White females were the primary recipient group" for ECT (p. 620). Qualitatively, it was apparent from the women's voices of the 1940s–1970s that psychiatric diagnosis and treatment were inextricably intertwined with family and gender roles (Showalter, 1985; Warren, 1987).

Women's voices were raised in protest over the diagnosis of women as insane and their treatment with ECT. Ollie Bozarth's critique of hospitalization and electroshock echoes in a more militant voice the words of the NAPA state hospital madwives fifteen years earlier: "Many husbands beat up their wives. . . . Other husbands just sign consent for the 'medical treatment' called shock, and let the experts do it for them. . . . Calling unusual, perhaps troublesome behavior an 'illness' allows any woman to be punished with psychiatric imprisonment, shock, psychosurgery, drugs, branding, loss of credibility. What a convenient way to control housewives who don't live up to the expectations of their husbands" (1976: 27). As Showalter put it in 1985, "In contemporary practice, medical management has replaced moral management as a way of containing women's suffering without confronting its causes" (p. 249).

Although both Warren (1987) and Showalter (1985) comment on the intersection of psychiatric and marital control in the mental hospitalization of women, they also note the flip side, "madness as a female strategy within the family" (Showalter, 1985: 246). Scholars have found in the madness of Roman, Enlightenment, Victorian, and twentieth-century women a form of protest against the duties and confinements of the female role. As Showalter said of one of R.D. Laing's female patients (1970): "The circumstances of her life, and particularly her marriage, made it difficult for Anna to be other than a patient. While she raised her two sons, David [her husband] put his energies into teaching and writing, and then into an extramarital affair. During one of her breakdowns, Anna jealously cried out to him, 'Yes you are a writer, and I am not creative, not grateful' " (Showalter, 1985: 242). The answer for Anna, as for many of the madwives of the 1950s, was mental hospitalization and electroshock.

MENTAL HEALTH LEGISLATION AND THE REGULATION OF ELECTROSHOCK

The efforts of the anti-shock activists—ex-patients, psychiatrists, religious ideologists and feminists—prompted legislative and regulatory action across America at the federal, state, and local level, and through both case and statutory law. Both patients' rights in general, and the right to refuse electroshock treatment specifically, were the targets of legislation. Prior to the 1960s, mental patients were considered wards of the state, and ECT was given without written consent. President Kennedy in 1963 issued a call for new legislation to protect the institutionalized (of which his sister Rosemary was one), and a new standard of patient care (Kennedy, 1964: 729–737). Federal policy also called for the "least restrictive environment" possible for mental patients, which served to limit institutionalization in some cases (Dain, 1989: 8), and the Community Mental Health Act mandated community care (Ewalt and Ewalt, 1969: 88).

Legislation at the federal and state level extended patients' rights during the late 1960s to early 1980s, regulating the involuntary commitment of mental patients to hospitals—one of the routes to ECT treatment (Warren, 1982). Constitutional protection for patients was at the core of the Supreme Court decision in *Wyatt v. Stickney* (1972). This important decision gave patients the right to informed consent. Prior to the late 1960s, mental patients were considered wards of the state, and ECT was given without consent. The Court in *Wyatt* held that mental patients had a right to treatment, a right to informed consent to treatment, a right to refuse treatment, a right to access their own patient records, and a right to due process in involuntary civil commitment (Starr, 1982: 389). In *Wyatt v. Hardin,* a follow-up decision to *Wyatt v. Stickney*, the Supreme Court refused to determine the medical applicability of ECT, but stressed specific patient rights and made recommendations for physicians who performed ECT (Winslade et al., 1984: 1350). The Minnesota Supreme Court singled out electroconvulsive therapy in the 1976 decision *Price v. Sheppard*, denying its use even on incompetent patients unless a court hearing showed cause for this treatment (Applebaum, 1994: 122). Utah in 1967 became the first state to regulate ECT (Slovenko, 1997: 523). Several states followed suit during the 1970s, including California and Massachusetts (Slovenko, 1997: 523; Grosser, 1975: 12–25; Clark and Lubenow, 1975: 86).

In 1979, Morrisey and his colleagues noted that "The legal limits on ECT have been barely explicated by court decisions. Beyond these the legal context of ECT relates to more generic case law dealing with the right to refuse treatment and statutory guidelines developed in California, New York, and Massachusetts, the three states with elaborated guidelines for the use of ECT" (p. 101). According to Morrisey, the three most "relevant" cases for ECT by 1978 were *Campbell v. Glenwood Hospital, Inc.* (1966), *Stein v. NYC Health and Hospitals Corporation* (1972), and *Wyatt v. Anderholt* (1977). In 1966 the courts found that ECT was a legitimate treatment for persons committed as "in need of care and treatment," while in 1972 they held that a patient could refuse ECT despite the fact that her mother consented. In the third case, the court decided that shock could not be classified as "just another somatic treatment" (Morrisey, Burton, and Steadman, 1979: 101). The right to refuse ECT was established, by 1980, only in California, New York, Massachusetts, North Carolina, and Wisconsin (Morrisey, Burton, and Steadman, 1979: 101).

The legal context for the right to refuse treatment, and statutory guidelines concerning the application of ECT, both involved questions of informed consent. The California legislature, under lobbying efforts by NAPA, passed State Assembly Bill AB 4481 in 1974, effective January 1, 1975. Among many other mandates, this bill required the patient's written informed consent to ECT, and that the treating physician's decision to use ECT be reviewed by three other physicians; furthermore it denied the treatment for all patients under age 12 (Winslade et al., 1984: 1351; Morrisey, Burton, and Steadman, 1979). Debates in Alabama and Michigan restricted ECT to use in state facilities, while the VA began to decrease the use of ECT in its hospitals (Fink, 1991: 795). By 1984, 37 states had some form of regulation concerning the use of ECT (Senter et al., 1984: 11).

ECT practitioners did not take the barrage of patients' rights and anti-ECT activism without protest; indeed, their own counteractivism was to some extent responsible for the later legislative turn back toward ECT (see Chapter 5). In California, Assemblyman Vasconcellos was criticized for his support of AB 4481, and various ECT specialists responded with indignation to the law. Allan M. Gunn-Smith of Stockton State Hospital in California complained about ECT's labeling by NAPA as "a bogus, barbaric, and destructive weapon," and about the inference that psychiatric professionals who administered it were "barbarians who get sadistic kicks out of punishing and torturing patients" (quoted in Friedberg, 1976: 176). Richard H. Trapnell of St. Francis Memorial Hospital in San Francisco "in a letter (dated Nov. 21, 1974) to the entire St. Francis medical staff found it 'deplorable that a small group [referring to NAPA] of ill-informed fanatics appear to have influenced Assemblyman Vasconcellos in sponsoring AB 4481' " (quoted in Breggin, 1979: 176). A decade later, Milton Greenblatt complained, "ECT: Please, No More Regulations!" in the *American Journal of Psychiatry*: "Understandable as manifestations of social anxiety but legally and clinically often without justification, excessive regulation and uninformed community uprisings contribute very little to enlightened decisionmaking" (1984b: 1410).

Other practitioners challenged mental health laws directly. In January 1975, two San Diego psychiatrists, Gary Aden and M. Brent Campbell, and one patient "Jane Doe," filed suit challenging the constitutionality of AB 4481 "on the basis that the bill infringed upon all psychiatric patients' rights to privacy and freedom of treatment" (Aden, 1975: 230). The psychiatrists claimed that the law was a "threat . . . to the patient receiving proper and timely treatment" by requiring unanimous consent of a panel of experts and trials of other treatments first. In an article based on statistical and case study follow-ups of pre- and post-AB 4481 ECT, Aden compared the "success" of the ECT-permitted with the "failure" of the ECT-denied cases:

Patient F, a 19-year-old Caucasian female, was treated conservatively for 90 [days] out of her 98-day hospitalization stay. During that time, she was evaluated for electrotherapy, beginning with the proposal for electrotherapy on the 75th day. Two consultants approved electrotherapy, while the third denied [it]. The dissenting consultant agreed to come back and take a look at the patient, and finally, under the patient's own insistence, was heard to tell the patient, "If you want your brains zapped, that's your business." The patient received electrotherapy and recovered from her withdrawn, reclusive state. The illness underwent a total remission. (Aden, 1975: 232)

In contrast, Patient A, a 29-year-old, Caucasian female "was rejected from electrotherapy . . . on the grounds that she did not fulfill the rigid criteria imposed by AB 4481. The patient . . . is 'simply on a plateau' " (Aden, 1975: 232). Aden and his colleagues also criticized AB 4481's consultant system, noting the age-old competition between physicians: "The very nature of consultation can result in a whimsical or faddish consultant utilizing his latest theory" (1975: 233). They argued that the denial of ECT led to longer hospitalizations than would have occurred without the treatment (Aden, 1975: 233). Finally, they asserted that restrictions on electroshock such as those embodied in AB 4481 were unnecessary in the face of the "natural attrition" of ECT in the 1970s (see below); this attrition, they claimed, countered critics' assertions that ECT was being abused (Aden, 1975: 233).

AB 4481 was struck down as unconstitutional by the state appeals court in 1978 on the following grounds: "(a) the requirement that the procedures be 'critically' needed was too ambiguous; (b) the patient's right to privacy was invaded by the stipulation that prior to treatment a responsible relative be informed concerning the items of informed consent; (c) review of choice of treatment by a review board was not necessary for competent patients; and (d) adequate hearings on the issues of competency and voluntariness were not provided" (Morrisey, Steadman, and Burton, 1979: 101–102). The substitute law, AB 1032, which became effective in 1977, "although still quite restrictive . . . did enable ECT to be given" (Kramer, 1985: 1190).

ELECTROSHOCK IN THE 1970s

Despite media and legislative attacks on ECT, the treatment continued to be used in psychiatric hospitals and on an outpatient basis during the 1970s. Clinical and survey research done during that time documents the age, gender, and race of patients, as well as the diagnoses for which the treatment was used, the number and duration of treatments, its successes and failures, and consent issues. Like many other studies, Morrisey and his colleagues in New York noted that the typical patient for ECT was "a relatively advantaged population of white, middle-class females whose treatment is covered by private insurance plans or other third parties" (1981: 618). Kramer concluded, similarly, that in California between 1977 and 1983 "far more white patients were given ECT than any other ethnic group" (p. 1191). Like earlier observers, he pointed out that 69 percent of ECT recipients were female, but claimed that "when adjusted for population [of mental hospitals] there was no difference in the incidence of ECT use among male and female patients" (p. 1190). For New York in 1972 and 1977, Morrisey and his colleagues found that the median age of ECT recipients in state facilities was 36 years, with an older population of recipients in other types of hospital— but with no mean age for any population higher than 55. Between 1977 and 1983, Kramer's (1985: 1192) California data indicate an aging of the ECT recipient population: there were 986 California ECT patients aged 65 and older, 894 aged 45–64, 655 aged 25–44, 114 aged 18–24, and 8 younger than 18 (see also Warren and Levy, 1991, and Chapter 5).

While ECT had been proposed mainly for serious psychotic and schizophrenic disorders in the early 1940s, by the 1970s the diagnostic emphasis had shifted to depressive disorders (Morrisey, Steadman, and Burton, 1981)— although there was a considerably diversity of diagnoses. Squire and his colleagues reported the following diagnoses among their 43 experimental ECT patients: severe depression (24 patients, including the diagnoses of psychotic depression, involutional melancholia, and primary affective disorder), depressive neurosis (6), schizoaffective disorder (5) and depressive neurosis (1). Patients with neurologic disorders or schizophrenia were excluded, as were alcoholics and drug users (1981: 89). In their 1975–1976 survey of New York ECT recipients in 30 facilities, Asnis, Fink, and Saferstein (1978) cited 12 diagnoses for which ECT was the treatment of choice, including endogenous depression (most patients), involutional depression (57 percent of patients), postpartum depression (50 percent), and anorexia nervosa (3 percent).

The number, duration, and conditions of treatment were also reported extensively in the clinical literature during the 1970s. In general, there was a decline from earlier decades in numbers of ECT patients and treatments, together with changes in practice such as the use of anesthesia and the placement of electrodes. In the Asnis, Fink, and Saferstein study, anesthesia was used for all treatments reported (1981: 480); this survey finding is not surprising given that anesthesia had been endorsed by the APA for the administration of ECT (Frankel, 1975: 77). In the 30 facilities studied by Asnis and his colleagues, 25 physicians used bilateral electrode placement exclusively, 2 used unilateral placement, and 3 used both types of placement (1978: 480). Squire and his colleagues used bilateral ECT with their 43 ECT recipients (1981: 89).

The 1970s clinical literature indicates that ECT was used less frequently and for a lesser duration than it had been during the 1950s–early 1960s. In Squire and his colleagues' study, ECT was administered "three times a week on alternate days after medication. . . . Treatments were given with 140 to 170 [volts]" (1981: 89). Total number of treatments for the experimental groups ranged from an average of 9.1 to an average of 13.6 (p. 90). Asnis and his colleagues (1978) reported that ECT was prescribed three times a week in 27 of the 30 New York facilities they surveyed, although some physicians gave four or five treatments per week. In the California hospital studied by Aden (1975), 60 patients received 657 treatments in 1974, while 36 patients received 364 treatments in 1975 (p. 231).

Research done in the 1970s explored the outcomes of ECT: cure and remission rates, the incidence of memory loss and other problems associated with the treatment, and informed consent issues. Scovern and Killman, in 1980, published a 40-page summary of the outcome literature on EST in America since the 1940s, including case history, experimental (using control groups with no treatment, sham shock, or alternative treatments), and retrospective studies. They concluded that "the pharmacological agents are inferior to ECT in reducing depressive symptomatology with endogenous depressives. With deluded or severely disturbed patients in this group, ECT is markedly superior to drug trials . . . the fast action of ECT makes it a preferred treatment when there is a risk of suicide in depressed patients" (1980: 298). These researchers concluded that ECT was less effective for schizophrenic, neurotic, or personality-disordered patients (1980: 298–299).

Not surprisingly, clinical studies of ECT starting from a position favorable to ECT treatment often presented favorable case studies of outcome (Aden, 1975, for example), while studies from the right-to-refuse treatment camp focused on problem cases (Friedberg, 1976, for example). Psychiatrists committed to ECT described the hazards of *not* treating, and highlighted the right to treatment. Salzman (1977) asked, rhetorically, "whether it is a physician's ethical right to *refuse* an effective treatment," and urged the reader to "Consider the following clinical vignette: A 49-year-old woman was voluntarily hospitalized with her third severe depression in 7 years.... Previous treatment with ECT at other institutions had offered rapid relief and a return of her ability to perform [as a concert violinist]. The patient refused antidepressant medication, which had made her more agitated in the past, and requested ECT. She denied memory loss from her previous treatments" (p. 1006).

Some research focused on the various complications of ECT, including the contested issue of short- or long-term memory loss. Studies of post-ECT memory loss are complicated by methodological issues. While some studies use tests of memory, such as lists of words, others use autobiographical memory as the source of information about ECT-induced memory loss. In their longitudinal study of 43 psychiatric patients treated with ECT, for example, Squire, Slater, and Miller (1981) used various forms of autobiographical memory, and the interview method, to study memory loss. They found that "(1) memory for remote events that occurred many years previously can initially be disrupted by bilateral ECT, but memory for these events appears to be fully recovered seven months later; (2) memory loss for events that occurred only a few days before treatment persisted; and (3) memory for events that occurred during the period one to two years before treatment was also vulnerable to ECT" (p. 95). These authors, cautiously, also pointed out that memory loss was far less with unilateral ECT, and that their overall "conclusion cannot be a strong one" given methodological problems of self-reported autobiographical memory (1981: 95).

Other complications of ECT were debated or studied in the 1970s literature, including health risks or death attendant upon either giving or denying ECT. Barry Kramer, in a public-statistics analysis of ECT in California between 1977 and 1983, noted that "the safety of ECT bears repeating. A death rate of 0.2 deaths/10,000 treatments is very low. . . . One can only guess at the number of patients who may have died because ECT was not available for them" (1985: 192). Clinical articles referred to careful consideration of contraindications for ECT, including brain tumors and myocardial infections (Asnis, Fink, and Saferstein, 1978: 480). By contrast, indications for ECT rather than psychoactive drugs were reported where the patient was pregnant or elderly (Warren and Levy, 1991).

Consent issues, another problem identified by the patients' rights and anti-psychiatry movements, was discussed in both the activist (pro and con) and ECT-survey and clinical literature. Kramer noted that "Involuntary ECT is a rarity in California; only 3 percent of the patients given ECT did not give their consent" (1985: 1191). In New York in 1975, Asnis and his colleagues claimed that "Written consent for ECT was obtained from each voluntary patient" in the 30 facilities they surveyed, but "procedures for patients who refused to consent differed and were poorly defined. Procedures varied from consent of a close relative to authorization of the treating physician and to strict requirement of a court order" (1978: 480). Warren and Levy (1991) found that documentation of written consent and other matters in involuntary ECT cases in Los Angeles was sparse during the late 1970s but increased during the early 1980s. Lidz and his colleagues describe the process by which informed consent was obtained in one hospital, Western Psychiatric, during the late 1970s–early 1980s:

> after having tried several drug combinations without success, the staff was urging [Ms. N] to consent to ECT. She told her [mental hospital] companions that, although she did not want to have ECT, she saw no other choice and repeatedly said, "If ECT doesn't work then I'll go to the bridge." For approximately a week, she struggled with the decision. . . . [She] had been given extensive information about it by staff members. . . . "You lie down and they give you an anesthetic and that relaxes you and then they put a little disc on one side of your head. It's unilateral not bilateral, and you go into a convulsion. I don't like the idea and I'm scared of it . . . because the doctors don't know a great deal about how it works and I'm scared because I don't want to lose my memory." . . . The other patients urged Ms. N to consent to ECT, telling her that it would help her and that the memory loss was only temporary. (Lidz, 1984: 150–151)

By 1979, Morrissey, Steadman, and Burton could conclude from the clinical and research literature in 1977–1978 that despite attacks on ECT "in both professional and lay circles," ECT had much to recommend it. They noted that "there is substantial evidence in support of ECT as an effective treatment in severe depressive illness." They suggested that electroshock was "superior" to pharmacological treatments such as tricyclids, "in terms of rapidity of response, discharge rate, length of hospitalization, and degree of symptomatic improvement" (p. 99). Yet despite this favorable review of ECT and others like it, the statistical evidence points to a decline in ECT use during the late 1960s and (at least the early) 1970s.

THE DECLINE OF ELECTROSHOCK

In the context of legislative and bureaucratic restrictions, unfavorable media publicity, scholarly critiques, the deinstitutionalization movement, psychopharmacology and insurance issues (see below), there was a steady decline in the use of electroshock in America during the 1960s and early 1970s (Katz, 1975; Aden, 1984c: 19). Since the treatment had most often been given on an inpatient basis in twentieth-century America, any decline in the number of inpatients in America would be likely to reduce the rate of treatment. Deinstitutionalization policies during the 1960s and early 1970s, although they might not have resulted in less restrictive "community care" for mental patients, did promote a shift from mental hospitalization to other forms of institutional care. In 1950, long-term hospitalization was one of the only options for institutionalization: 39 percent of all institutionalized persons were in mental hospitals in comparison to 17 percent in correctional facilities and 19 percent in nursing homes. By 1960 the percentage of institutionalized persons in mental hospitals had fallen to 33 percent; nursing home placement had increased to 25 percent and correctional to 18 percent. In 1970, 20 percent of institutionalized persons were in mental hospitals, 15 percent in correctional facilities, and 44 percent in nursing homes, reflecting the aging of the American population (Kramer, 1977). Since ECT is a treatment associated with psychiatric hospitalization rather than other forms of institutional care, its patient base decreased to the extent that mental patients were de- or trans-institutionalized.

Numerous studies were done during the 1970s to determine the use of ECT in various settings. These studies were necessary because the reporting of ECT treatments to federal agencies such as NIMH was, by the mid-1970s, mandated only in a patchwork manner: required, for example, for federal Veterans Administration hospitals, but not for private psychiatric hospitals. Only California, from 1977 on, mandated the reporting of all ECT to the Sacramento Office of Patients' Rights, thus the only close-to-complete data on ECT we have for the 1970s comes from that state. Other studies rely on surveys of local hospitals, with all the methodological problems, including response rate, attendant upon survey research. In addition, it is often mainly metropolitan areas such as New York that have the funds and personnel available for such surveys (see, for example, Asnis, Fink, and Saferstein, 1978; Morrisey, Steadman, and Burton, 1979; 1981). Case studies of single hospitals were also done during the 1970s, such as the work of Aden (1975) in California.

With these caveats in mind, there are several studies that document the decline of ECT at the local or national level. In their study of the "natural attrition" of the use of ECT in their California hospital prior to the passage of AB 4481, Aden and his colleagues claimed a 50 percent reduction, from 2,171 inpatients and 371 outpatients in 1968 to 1,201 inpatients and 139 outpatients in 1974 (Aden, 1975: 231). In contrast to Warren and Levy (1991), Kramer (1985) asserted that the availability of ECT "steadily declined" in California from 1977–1983. In a New York state survey, Morrisey and his colleagues found that there was a 40.2 percent decline in ECT use between 1972 and 1977 (1979: 108). Tellingly, while these authors cited a "long-term decline in ECT use," they also commented that the six for-profit general hospitals in their samples experienced a 129 percent growth in the number of ECT patients (Morrisey, Steadman, and Burton, 1981: 619; and see below).

At the national level, Greenblatt (1977) argued that by the mid-1970s, there was a decrease in the use of ECT nationwide by 90 percent in state hospitals and 33 percent in reporting private hospitals. A 1975 survey by the National Institute of Mental Health, based on admissions to mental hospitals and discharges from general hospitals with psychiatric units, indicated an overall estimate of 60,000 cases of ECT, or 8.5 percent of the total treated psychiatrically (Morrisey, Burton, and Steadman, 1979: 102). Thompson and Blaine (1987: 557–558) documented a 46 percent decline in the use of ECT in America in all types of hospital between 1975 and 1980; the rate of ECT treatments per 100,000 patients in private general hospitals went from 27.5 percent in 1975 to 14.7 percent in 1980.

By 1980, the rate of ECT was lowest in state psychiatric hospitals (Thompson and Blaine, 1987: 558). State hospitals were either forbidden to provide the treatment, or, like the VA hospital system, so hampered by bureaucratic red tape that the treatment was, in effect, not available. In 1975, state and county hospitals treated only 1 percent of their patients with ECT (Morrisey, Burton, and Steadman, 1979: 102); by 1980, of the 159,000 admissions to VA hospitals, only 526 patients were treated with ECT (Isaac and Armat, 1990: 205).

Private hospitals, as they would continue to be in the 1980s and 1990s (see Chapter 5), became the primary site of ECT treatments (Fink, 1979: 16; Morrisey, Steadman, and Burton, 1979: 102), although the statistics on private-hospital ECT may be skewed by the intensive usage of a few of them (Morrisey, Steadman, and Burton, 1979: 108). Of the total ECT cases in a 1973–1974 Massachusetts survey, 90 percent were in private mental hospitals, 6 percent in state hospitals, and 4 percent in VA hospitals (Morrisey, Steadman, and Burton, 1979: 102). In New York in a 1975–1976 survey, the percentage of patients receiving ECT was 1 percent for public facilities, 5 percent for private nonprofit university-affiliated facilities, and 21 percent for admissions to private proprietary hospitals (Morrisey, Burton, and Steadman, 1979: 102–103). By 1979, Morrisey, Burton, and Steadman concluded that "ECT use is much more prevalent in private as opposed to public facilities" and "has undergone a dramatic decline in recent years" (p. 109).

A 1980 summary of the incidence of ECT in American private psychiatric hospitals came to the same conclusion about public vs. private hospitals, but a different one about the decline of ECT. Noting that the distribution of ECT was quite uneven depending upon geographical locale as well as type of hospital, psychiatrist Robitscher (1980: 277) noted that some private proprietary (for-profit) hospitals treated from 50–70 percent of patients with ECT. A survey of the practice in 36 metropolitan New York mental hospitals indicated that 13 shocked 1–5 percent, 7 shocked 6–15 percent, and 4 shocked 16–40 percent. One "famous psychiatric hospital, not run for profit" reported a yearly rate of 7.5 percent ECT treatments for inpatients (Robitscher, 1980: 277). It is clear that the seeds of the private-hospital expansion of ECT during the 1980s–1990s (see Chapter 5) were planted during the era of ECT's decline, and that some of these seeds were economic.

Besides trends toward deinstitutionalizing mental patients and legislation aimed at expanding patients' rights, there were economic factors in the 1960s–1970s that affected ECT usage. These included the cost of shock machines and procedures, malpractice insurance, and third-party payment policies. The economic complexity of ECT during the 1960s–1970s was reflected in the changing technology and availability of the ECT machine. In the 1940s some physicians made their own machines or brought them from Europe; by 1970 the machines themselves had become more elaborate and costly, and less widely available. Offner sold his company in the 1950s and the new owners stopped manufacturing EST devices (Lewis and Ray, 1984: 35). "Virtually the only U.S. manufactured device" in 1970 was the Medcraft B24 Mark III (Stephans, Greenberg, and Pettinati, 1991: 1004). Psychiatrists who used EST were forced to use older models; the American Psychiatric Association's task force report on EST found that 67 percent of EST practitioners used Medcraft, another 33 percent used Reiter, and another 1 percent the newest line, MECTA (American Psychiatric Association, 1978: 6–7), invented by psychiatrist Paul Blachly in 1973. In addition, recommendations or mandates for sedation and anesthesia added to the hospital and outpatient costs and inconveniences. These "hidden costs" to physicians for ECT use included the requirement that the treatment (unlike drugs) be administered by a physician rather than a nurse. The physician's workload might increase by using ECT, since the treatment generally resulted in higher patient turnover.

During this era, economic as well as clinical factors shaped the choice for or against ECT in the context of different types of hospital organization and financing. In private hospitals, physicians were usually paid on a fee-for-service basis; the financial compensation received for giving ECT may have offset the necessity of additional work and inconvenience. Similarly, private hospitals themselves were usually reimbursed for each service rendered. Thus, it was to the mutual advantage of both hospital and physician to set up psychiatric wards conducive to the use of ECT. Yet in the public hospitals "neither the salaried staff physicians nor the hospital are paid additionally for ECT. Lack of necessary equipment, ancillary staff, additional physician workload and inconvenience may result. [In] University hospitals . . . the salaried professor of psychiatry is able to make a clinical decision to use ECT without being influenced by the inconvenience or the potential profit associated with delivering the treatment" (Bailine and Rau, 1981: 279). The expense of delivering ECT led one municipal hospital, faced with cutting costs in the poor economy of the 1970s, to eliminate ECT by removing "the funds for the anesthesiologist" (Asnis, Fink, and Saferstein, 1978: 481).

Malpractice insurance became more problematic for psychiatrists during the 1960s and 1970s, although malpractice suits concerning ECT were few and the awards minimal (Fink and Bailine, 1998: 110). Even though most malpractice cases were based on the improper administration of ECT and the average out-of-court settlement only a little over a thousand dollars (Appelbaum, 1994: 522), higher premiums were required from ECT practitioners, leading Milton Greenblatt to call them "excessive" (Greenblatt, 1984a: 4). As one observer commented, "A psychiatrist, giving as few as one ECT a year, can find his professional liability insurance four times that of a non-ECT using colleague" (Callan, 1979: 545; see also Hyde, 1975: 46). Anecdotal reports by practitioners suggest that increases in malpractice insurance rates led to a decline in the number of psychiatrists willing to give ECT (*Convulsive Therapy Bulletin* 1975: 6; Hay, 1989: 5). For example, ECT pioneer Lothar Kalinowsky (1982) gave maintenance ECT in his office for thirty years but finally abandoned ambulatory ECT in the face of malpractice insurance costs for his anesthesiologist. His experience was not isolated (Slovenko, 1997: 524).

The 1960s–1970s also saw changes in third-party insurance practices. At the same time as the federal government was revamping the location of mental health treatment through the Community Mental Health Act, plans were being formulated for a national insurance program. Picking up where Kennedy had left off, President Lyndon Johnson sponsored legislation that eventually became the Social Security Amendments of 1965, creating Title 18 (better known as Medicare) and Title 19 (better known as Medicaid) (Stevens and Stevens, 1974: 46). Medicare was designed to provide health insurance to the aged, while Medicaid was aimed at families with dependent children as well as "the blind or permanently disabled" (Stevens and Stevens, 1974: 57).

Psychiatrists faced restrictions on billings, while Medicaid and Blue Shield limited the amount of funding per treatment (Hyde, 1975: 46). In the 1970s, Blue Cross limited the number of days of hospitalization, 30 days for psychiatric patients as opposed to the standard 125 for all other major illnesses (Grob, 1991: 268). In the period from 1965 to 1980, Medicare limited payments to state institutions and outpatient psychiatric services, and excluded psychiatric payments for patients in general hospitals. Medicaid "specifically excluded financial support for mental hospital patients under the age of 65" (Grob 1991: 268). A study of ECT in California reflects the economic reality of ECT. Patients who received the treatment between 1977 and 1983 paid out of pocket 30 percent of the time and used their third-party insurance 25 percent of the time, while another 37 percent of patients were covered under the California (Short-Doyle) or federal insurance (Medicaid, Medicare) plans (Kramer, 1985: 1190–1191).

By the early 1970s, the death knell for ECT seemed to be sounding. Pressured by health-care costs, undercut by the growth of psychopharmacology, thwarted by the imagery of *Cuckoo's Nest* and the vast cultural, legal, economic, and political changes of the late 1960s, it's not surprising that one midcentury psychiatrist wondered, "Is Shock Treatment Becoming Obsolete?" (Wortis, 1962) while another predicted that the widespread practice of ECT "will not last another 40 years, nor indeed to the end of the century. Perhaps even by the end of this decade, electroconvulsive therapy for severely depressed states will be replaced by more effective and selective drugs" (Palmer, 1981: 2).

But the demise of ECT, unlike its electrotherapeutic predecessors, was not to be. During the late 1970s the tide had already begun to turn with California statistics showing the start of what was to be a decades-long increase in ECT treatments in the state (Warren and Levy, 1991). As early as 1980, one psychiatrist noted that "shock is very advantageous" economically for hospitals (Robitscher, 1980: 278)—if not necessarily for individual psychiatrists. By that time, many health-care policies would only pay for three weeks of inpatient psychiatric care—"just the right period to complete a course of eight treatments" according to anti-ECT psychiatrist Robitscher, who implied that some hospitals were quasi-ECT mills "that give electroshock treatment to almost all of their patients regardless of the diagnosis." These hospitals were often very profitable because "in addition to money received from private insurance companies, government funds pay for treatment given to Medicare, Medicaid, and other patients" (Robitscher, 1980: 278–279). In the context of economic as well as cultural and political forces during this era, the stage was set for the rebirth of ECT after its brief decline.

Chapter 5

Pushbutton Triumphant: The Rebirth of Electroshock, 1981–1999

A 74-year-old grandmother and retired bookkeeper wearing street clothes and makeup was being prepared for a procedure that doctors hoped would end a depression so severe that she had practically stopped eating. After she received muscle relaxants and mild barbiturates, a doctor applied electrodes to her temple. In minutes she was asleep. As "It's Only a Paper Moon" wafted from a speaker nearby, the doctor pushed a button on a gray box releasing two seconds of electric current, for about 45 seconds, her arms and legs jerked a few inches up and down, her expression did not change.

—Lisa Foderaro, 1993

ECT, already moving toward rehabilitation by the late 1970s, reemerged in the 1980s and 1990s as "the gold standard antidepressant treatment modality" (Zimmer and Price, 1991: 439). By the closing decade of the twentieth century American psychiatry had moved once again toward somatic explanations and treatments for mental illness. Some scientists had mapped the human genome, foregrounding genetic explanations for human social behavior, while others sought their etiologies in fluids—no longer the humors, but the hormones. Repudiating a psychiatry based on the authority of the therapist, somatic psychiatrists concurred that "The old psychiatry derives from theory, the new psychiatry from fact" (Kirk and Krutchins, 1992: 7). Somaticists dominated the academy, holding, from 1975 on, the most numerous and important positions in medical schools (Grob, 1994: 277). Returning from twenty years in Brazil, one American-trained psychiatrist was shocked to find "A whole new generation of psychiatrists coming from the best medical schools trained in the best American mechanistic and pragmatic tradition" (quoted in Breggin, 1991: 16).

This shift toward somaticism was marked by the publication of the third edition of the *Diagnostic and Statistical Manual (DSM)* of the APA in 1980 and the fourth in 1994. In these editions, the *DSM* shifted its emphasis from psychological to biological explanations (Kirk and Krutchins, 1992: 7), the

Food and Drug Administration (FDA) declaring, in the late 1990s, that "Study after study suggest[s] biochemical and genetic links to depression" (Nordenberg, 1998: n.p.). Continuing psychiatry's expansionary and scientific quest, *DSM* III and IV also specified and elaborated in ever-growing detail the symptomatology of an ever-growing number of mental disorders.

The return of somaticism fostered both pharmacology and ECT, while the limits of pharmacology facilitated the turn to ECT. From the 1950s to the 1970s drugs in general, and particularly new drugs, had captured the public imagination as "magic bullets" that would finally conquer mental illness. One of these substances, Prozac, became so widely prescribed and disseminated throughout the inpatient and outpatient population that America was labeled the *Prozac Nation* (Wurtzel, 1994). Each of the new drugs after its first "honeymoon" period caused problems, including the effects that medicine calls "side." These ranged from discomforts such as weight gain, dry mouth, or sleep disturbance—associated with antidepressants such as Elavil—to the Parkinson's-like tardive dyskinesia sometimes caused by neuroleptics or major tranquilizers (Klein and Wender, 1995: 132–133). Far from a "magic bullet" preventing depression and suicide, some psychiatric and media depictions of Prozac asserted that the drug *caused* suicide (Breggin, 1995: 150–151).

Side effects, tolerance, and other medical problems associated with the use of psychoactive drugs set the stage for the return of ECT, as did the social problems related to deinstitutionalization and the war on drugs. According to one historian of psychiatry, the rhetoric of the war on illegal drugs during the 1980s spilled over into the arena of prescription drugs; by the 1980s, "tranquilizers, along with many other psychoactive drugs, had become almost demonized" (Speaker, 1997: 356). The "human rights" rhetoric of deinstitutionalization had changed, by the 1980s, to one of "throwing helpless (or dangerous) mental patients out into the street" without benefit of real community care (Grob, 1994: 300–302). Some psychiatrists, health-care workers, and even patients' rights advocates argued that ECT was a benefit society arbitrarily denied the mentally ill (Andreasen, 1984: 108).

Throughout the 1960s, ECT had been used for the treatment of affective disorders. And the last two decades of the twentieth century were characterized by mental health experts as the "Age of Melancholy" (Schrof and Schultz, 1999: 56–57), in which diagnoses of depression had doubled since World War II. The World Health Organization predicted that by 2020 depression would be the world's second most disabling disease, suggesting that by 1999 it was already *the* most disabling illness for women (Schrof and Schultz, 1999: 56). In the wake of fifty years of prescribing psychoactive drugs for depression, drugs to which some patients were tolerant or resistant, ECT was once again proposed as the most effective treatment for depression (Banzak, 1996: 273). And, as we shall see below, the growing population of elderly depressed patients had, by the 1990s, become the primary target of ECT.

The return of electroshock recapitulated some of the contexts surrounding the initial dissemination of ECT in America: a purported "crisis" in mental health care, a rejection of Freudian psychotherapy accompanying a somatic turn in psychiatry, and the perceived failure of other treatment modalities. During the 1980s–1990s there were economic contingencies—particularly the structuring of public and private insurance—that facilitated the return of electroshock, especially in private and for-profit hospitals. And, as in the earlier eras of ECT, psychiatric, state, and federal organizations debated and lobbied for the regulation or deregulation of ECT.

THE ORGANIZATIONAL POLITICS OF ELECTROSHOCK

During the 1970s and 1980s, pro-ECT psychiatrists strove to rehabilitate the treatment at the local and national levels. In 1972 Milton Greenblatt, by then State Commissioner for Mental Health in Massachusetts, formed a task force on ECT chaired by Fred Frankel of Harvard (Shorter, 1997: 294). This group developed by 1975 into the task force on ECT within the APA, issuing its first report in 1978 (Frankel, 1978). Also in 1975, the International Psychiatric Association for the Advancement of Electrotherapy (IPAAE) formed, adopting *Convulsive Therapy and Tardive Dyskinesia Notes* as its official organ; this group later became the Association for Convulsive Therapy (Aden, 1984b: 9–10). Working with the APA, the IPAAE filed a brief as "friends of the court" to fight the 1982 Berkeley ban on ECT, which it succeeded in overturning (Clark, Schmidt, and Hagar, 1982: 105; Herbert, 1982: 309; Herbert, 1983: 71; Greenblatt, 1984: 4). But the crucial organizational battle over the "new" ECT occurred between 1979 and 1987, when pro- and anti-ECT psychiatrists clashed over attempts by the "antis" to make the federal government the ultimate ECT watchdog.

In 1976 Congress mandated that the FDA regulate medical devices. The Bureau of Medical Devices, an FDA subcommittee, proposed in April 1978 the reclassification of ECT machinery from a Class II device (one that requires "performance standards"), to a Class III device (one that involves "unreasonable risk for injury or illness" and must therefore follow higher criteria for certification by the FDA). Reclassification was prompted by the Advisory Panel on Neurological Devices within the Medical Devices office of the FDA. The neurologists cited brain damage and memory loss as issues of concern with the use of ECT machines. At hearing of this panel held in 1977 Linda Purdue of the Church of Scientology's Commission on Human Rights testified that ECT machines caused brain damage. ECT proponent Richard Weiner represented the newly created APA task force on ECT, and Harry Feinstein, a representative of the Hittman Corporation, one of the few manufacturers of ECT devices, spoke in favor of the machines (Farber, 1995: 150). Manufacturers had a strong incentive to battle the reclassification; one FDA official estimated that if manufacturers had to pre-market test their machines their costs would increase by more than three million dollars (Isaac and Armat: 1990: 209).

Psychiatrists reacted strongly to what Dr. Melvin Sabshin, medical director of the APA, called the "neurological bias" in the panel membership (Joint Information Services Files, 1979: I). Claiming that the APA's decision was a response to "vocal anti-psychiatric individuals and groups, Peter Breggin among them," the APA portrayed the FDA decision as an intrusion of nonprofessionals into psychiatric domains, singling out "Breggin's stable of ex-patients." Depicting psychiatry as under siege, the APA mobilized its members, who were told that "everywhere we are losing the battle" (Joint Information Services Files, 1980, II). The APA even suggested legal action as a means of muting anti-ECT opposition, noting that "It might be appropriate that our legal counsel study the books and testimony of the anti-ECT and anti-psychiatric groups to determine if any statements were libelous and likely to deprive APA members of their legitimate livelihoods. If so, would a lawsuit be warranted and would it be useful in inhibiting such irresponsible and destructive activities?" (Joint Information Services Files, 1980: I). The APA did not, in the end, sue anyone for libel, but it did pursue a variety of avenues for the rehabilitation of ECT during the 1980s. After the FDA decision to reclassify the devices, the APA requested that further hearings be held prior to implementation (Weck, 1986: 9–11).

The FDA approved the APA's petition, and further hearings were held in November, 1982. In a well-orchestrated demonstration, Richard Weiner gathered a number of patients to speak on behalf of ECT and counter the negative impact of patients opposed to it (Joint Information Services, 1982: I). Within the APA, internal memos debated whether the organization should use its newsletter, *Psychiatric News*, to mobilize members. One member concluded: "I don't think we should urge members to write in [to the FDA] as it smacks of an organized campaign which might have a negative impact" (Joint Information Services, 1984: I).

Following the 1982 hearings, the FDA delayed the decision to move ECT to Class III devices and maintained them under the guidelines of Class II (Isaac and Armat, 1990: 208). A new relationship between the APA and FDA began after 1982 as the APA cooperated with the FDA in negotiating a number of issues regarding the use of ECT machines. The FDA accepted the established criterion of existing ECT machines as meeting the required "performance standards" necessary for Class II medical devices. In the 1990s conflict between the two organizations resurfaced over attempts by the FDA to limit ECT use with patients suffering from schizophrenia or mania, attempts that were thwarted by the APA (Fink, 1991: 796). Electroshock proponents, who generally sought improved energy levels in ECT devices, were also concerned that the "arbitrary" requirement that older machines meet performance standards limited the modification capabilities of the machines. Patients, who build up convulsive resistance thresholds over time, require larger amounts of energy to reach convulsion (Sakeim, 1991: 233–236).

Proponents of ECT found support, during the 1980s and 1990s in the federal government, beginning with the National Institute for Mental Health (NIMH). In 1985 the NIMH held a Consensus Conference on ECT and a panel consisting of health professionals, a lawyer, and a consumer advocate, and chaired by Robert Rose of the University of Texas, met for three days in Maryland to hear testimony for and against ECT. The conference panel not only endorsed ECT (Holden, 1985: 1510–1511; Bower, 1985: 389), but the NIMH turned to the APA to write additional guidelines for the use of shock. This led to the creation, in 1987, of a permanent committee on ECT within the APA, which subsequently sought funding from NIMH. The partnership between APA and NIMH resulted in *The Second Task Force Report on ECT*, a document that included indications for the use of shock as a first line of treatment rather than as a last resort (Weiner et al., 1990). In 1999 the surgeon general released a report on mental health that included a favorable assessment of the role of ECT.

A 1980s–1990s campaign to win over other psychiatrists to ECT began with the publication of several new textbooks on ECT, including the leading text published by Dr. Richard Abrams in 1982. ECT was also given favorable press in special issues of professional journals, such as a 1984 issue of the *American Journal of Social Psychiatry* and a 1991 issue of the *Psychiatric Clinics of North America*. In the 1991 issue, the editor declared that "there is no scientific controversy about ECT" (Kellner, 1991: 1). Apparently the AMA concurred; in 1989 its House of Delegates passed a resolution supporting ECT.

In 1985, Max Fink—a protégé of Lothar Kalinowsky—became the recognized leader of ECT studies when he launched *Convulsive Therapy*, later *The Journal of ECT*, to serve the "renewed interest" of the medical profession in ECT; the journal served as the official publication of the Convulsive Therapy Association, formed in 1984 to promote research and disseminate information on shock. Fink had been active in the research and promotion of electroshock since the early 1950s, and served at the State University of New York at Stony Brook from 1972 to 1997. Fink's impact on twentieth-century American psychiatry was second only to Lothar Kalinowsky's, and he is credited by medical historian Edward Shorter with the return of ECT to respectability in the 1980s (Shorter, 1998: 45). When Fink retired as editor of *Convulsive Therapy* in 1993 he was succeeded by Dr. Charles Kellner.

The renewed interest in ECT in the 1980s was reflected in an increasing number of scholarly articles and popular pieces. The Menninger clinic, for example, called ECT an "old therapy that brings new hope" in a 1991 issue of the *Menninger Perspective*. Both professional and popular treatments of ECT sang its praises and minimized its dangers: "Over the past 50 years,

ECT has evolved into a state-of-the art medical procedure far removed from its original, rather primitive, form" (Weiner and Krystal, 1994: 280). The psychiatric literature, from 1980 onward, dismissed as methodologically flawed earlier studies that warned of side effects. These studies were described as "not careful," with ECT proponents arguing that "little evidence" existed to back up such "side effects" as "memory impairment [of] six to nine months or longer" (Karasu, 1984: 230). One text claimed that there was "no evidence of any long-term effect on learning or memory," and that "ECT is probably the safest and most effective treatment available for depressive illness" (Andreasen, 1984: 108).

Pro-ECT texts in the 1980s–1990s proposed theories of causation similar to those of earlier decades. There was virtual unanimity that it was not the electricity that caused the physical changes leading to remission of symptoms, but the convulsion (but see O'Brien, 1989). Some 1980s–1990s ECT practitioners still viewed the treatment as an empirical one: it works, but we do not know how it works (Manning, 1995). Max Fink himself confessed that "we simply don't understand how ECT has the restorative capacity that it does" (Fink, 2000: 163). 1990s theories of electroshock's operation were overwhelmingly somatic, including chemical theories of neurotransmitter or neuroendocrine changes induced by the seizure (Cauchon, 1995: 9). In some of this literature, hormones such as dopamine and serotonin (Manning, 1995; Abrams, 1986) took the center stage once occupied by the humors (see Chapter 1). Changes in the brain were also proposed as the mechanism for electroshock's effect: "brain stimulation" for pro-ECT psychiatrists (Pearlman, 1991: 133) and "brain damage" for those opposed (Breggin, 1995). Even the Hippocratics-to-Meduna proposal (see Chapters 1 and 3) that induced seizures were incompatible with mental illness reappeared in the 1990s as the anti-convulsant theory: "Shock-induced seizures teach the brain to resist seizures. This effort to resist seizures dampens abnormally active brain circuits, stabilizing mood" (Cauchon, 1995: 9). Mechanistic imagery also reemerged in the 1980s in popular depictions of ECT; in one best-selling novel a doctor explained that "electroconvulsive treatment or ECT is the equivalent of rebooting a computer" (Cornwell, 1991: 284).

The popular print media published a number of pieces favorable to ECT during the late 1970s to mid-1990s. An article in the *New York Times Magazine* compared the treatment to "wizardry" (1979), while *Time* heralded the "comeback of ECT" (1979), and *Science Digest* (1984) stressed the new, more "patient friendly" technologies of ECT. *Psychology Today*, once a forum for opponents of ECT, claimed that the treatment was not only safe and effective, but it was underused (1995). Ironically, some who supported the return of ECT charged the media with responsibility for its earlier demise: "The reluctance of patients and doctors to accept the fact that ECT is safe and effective is a sad commentary on the power of the media to influence our perceptions" (Andreasen, 1984: 108). Both the media and the anti-psychiatry movements were dismissed by one historian of psychiatry as "neo-romantics" (Dain, 1989: 2–12), although by the mid-1990s, articles critical of shock began once more to appear in the media (for example, Cauchon, 1995).

THE TECHNOLOGIES AND ECONOMICS OF ECT

Part of the rehabilitation of ECT during the 1980s and 1990s was premised upon pro-ECT practitioners' and ECT manufacturers' claims that both the machinery and the procedures used in contemporary shock were very different than those of the 1940s–1950s—"more humane" (using sedatives and anesthesia), safer, more effective, and without brutalizing effects such as broken limbs. Companies that made ECT machines—MECTA, Somatics, Medcraft, and Elcot—equipped their most expensive 1990s models with computer enhancements that suggested greater control and more exact science. These features incorporated a variety of monitoring devices such as EEGs (electroencephalograms) and EKGs (electrocardiograms), both of which were used by psychiatrist Paul Blachly when he invented the MECTA (Monitored Electro Convulsive Therapy Apparatus) in the early 1970s (Lewis and Ray, 1984: 35), and "brain mapping computers" that "monitor the currents and direct the shocks to only one side of the head" (Gelman et al., 1987: 52).

There is no doubt that the technology of the machine had changed since the "black boxes" of the 1940s, when some psychiatrists (like those of earlier centuries) built their own machines. But the exact nature and medical worth of those changes were still, by the end of the twentieth century, the subject of controversies between opponents and practitioners of ECT. The proponents and manufacturers of ECT machines claimed that the treatment was safer than in the 1950s because of the use of unilateral rather than bilateral electrode placement, shorter bursts of electricity, and less electricity (Fink, 1999). Opponents, however, counterclaimed that the new ECT machines actually used more energy (ranges up to 500 volts) than in earlier decades when they used around 120 volts (Cameron, 1994: 192), or could cause greater damage to more carefully localized areas (Eastgate, 1998: 30; Cameron, 1994: 193). Although sedatives and anesthesia were routinely used by the 1990s, they were not used universally—and patients might (Lehmann, 1982), or might not find these additions more humane. One 69-year-old woman who had ECT in the late 1970s said that she "hated it" and "I especially don't like the anesthesia. I lose control" (Warren and Levy, 1991: 319).

The economics of ECT were also relevant to its rehabilitation. These economics occurred at several points: ties between ECT psychiatrists and machine- and video-making corporations; money made from administering the treatment; the intersection of insurance with hospital and outpatient organizations; and costs of the treatment to providers. All but the cost of the treatment to providers—which included capital outlay, provision of staff, and malpractice insurance—fostered rather than retarded the growth of ECT during the last decades of the twentieth century.

There were close ties between ECT psychiatrists and ECT video and machine manufacturers during the 1980s–1990s. MECTA was the invention of psychiatrist Paul Blachly, one of the founders of the International Association for the Advancement of Electrotherapy in 1975 (Cameron, 1994: 190). Some members of the American Psychiatric Association Task Force on ECT were also linked fiscally to the manufacturers of ECT devices. Richard Abrams and Conrad Swartz began Somatics in 1985 (Stephans et al., 1991: 989), a company which sold more than half of all ECT machines in the 1990s; in the late 1990s Somatics sales reached a million dollars (Neoforma, 1999). Richard Abrams, the author of the leading text on ECT (1992), derived more than 50 percent of his income from the company (Eastgate, 1998: 30; Cauchon, 1995: 6).

Videotapes of ECT procedures were prepared by manufacturers and practitioners to counter the imagery of death and punishment portrayed in *One Flew Over the Cuckoo's Nest*, and replace it with scenes of rebirth and renewal. MECTA created a video for professionals that featured Richard Weiner and Harold Sackeim, while Somatics hired both Sackeim and Max Fink to prepare its videos. Fink received $18,000 for his work and 8 percent royalty on the $350 videos (Boorman 1996: 14; Cameron, 1994: 181). One critic of the intersection of the professional, organizational, and technological with the economics of ECT remarked that the APA Task Force on Psychiatry ought to be called "The Manufacturers' Task Force Report on ECT" (Cameron, 1994: 181).

As we indicated in the last chapter, the locus of ECT treatment was, by 1980, the private or teaching rather than the public hospital; this trend continued into the 1980s and 1990s. By 1988, the number of American private hospitals providing ECT had risen to 444, from only 48 in 1970. Both physicians and patients (as well as the hospitals themselves) benefited economically from the turn to ECT, according to a number of studies. Private hospital psychiatrists were able to make $27,000–$30,000 per year just for being in attendance at ECT treatments (Eastgate, 1998: 30; Cauchon, 1985: 3). Psychiatrists' fees were anywhere from $125 to $250 for the 5- to 15-minute procedure (Cauchon, 1995: 3); a study published in 1998 found that Medicare paid $97.73 and Medicaid $36 for psychiatrists attending ECT, the anesthesiologist's fees ranged from $75 to $160, while the nurse and treatment room added another $500 per treatment (Fink and Bailine, 1998: 110).

Despite these costs, according to pro-ECT publications, patients (and insurance companies) saved money, from both shorter hospital stays (APA 1998: 20–22) and the comparative cost of ECT and psychopharmacology. A course of tricyclids in the hospital was estimated at $26,481 in 1998, and a course of ECT at $20,079 (Fink and Bailine, 1998: 110). In 1998, ambulatory or outpatient ECT was estimated to be considerably less expensive than inpatient, about $531 per treatment or $4,350 per course (Bailine, 1998: 256). Anti-ECT publications pointed out that the costs of the treatment were still high. According to anti-ECT journalist Cauchon (1995: 3), the costs for one shock at a Sacramento, California hospital were: $175 for the psychiatrist; $300 for the anesthesiologist; and $375 for the use of the hospital's shock therapy room. One patient "received a total of 21 shocks, costing about $18,000. The hospital charged another $890 a day for her room. Private insurance paid."

Part of the economic context of private hospitals' renewed provision of ECT in the 1980s–1990s had to do with insurance, both public and private. Public insurance—Medicare, Medicaid, and Supplemental Social Security Income—had a profound and complex impact on hospitals during the 1970s–1980s (Starr, 1982) much of which is beyond the scope of this discussion. A *USA Today* journalist, albeit cynically, highlighted the impact of public insurance on the provision of ECT in Texas hospitals: "65-year-olds get 360 percent more shock therapy than 64-year-olds. The difference: Medicare pays" (Cauchon, 1995: 1). This was also the conclusion of another journalist who claimed that Medicare had become the single biggest source of reimbursement for ECT and that it paid more for ECT treatment than for psychotherapy (Boodman, 1996).

The ways in which private insurance paid for medical treatments, and the treatments they paid for, changed many times during the twentieth century; these changes, in turn, affected the provision of somatic or psychological therapies. Reductions in the length of hospital stays reimbursed by private insurance during the 1980s, for example, set time limits on trials of psychoactive drugs. The advent of diagnostic related groups (DRGs) in the 1980s also changed psychiatric practice; as the March 1985 *APA Monitor* commented: "Cynical observers have noted that the advent of diagnostic related groups (DRGs) for hospital reimbursement may make ECT more cost-effective than drugs. It works 30 to 40 percent faster, according to at least one study" (p. 18).

The consensus among observers of the mental health system, including psychiatrists, seemed to be that economic factors were important in the resurgence of ECT in the 1980s. Although expensive in malpractice insurance and initial capital outlay, ECT was cheap and rapid in actual administration (Robitscher, 1980). A psychiatrist interviewed by Warren in 1988 said that "economic factors are the most important in the rise of ECT—I sound like a Marxist—especially since January. Medicare will now pay up to $1,000 in outpatient psychiatric care bills rather than the $200 or so they paid before. The economics of these situations determine the treatments. If Medicare paid for longer hospitalizations the psychiatrists might be willing to go through more drug series to see if they worked." He also noted that "adding ECT to a private practice is an expensive business that adds $2,000–$3,000 per year to malpractice insurance costs." This figure, however, represented considerably less than malpractice surcharges of the 1960s and 1970s (Aden, 1984b: 10).

ECT PATIENTS: GENDER AND AGE

During the 1980s–1990s, more women than men were ECT recipients—but, increasingly, not as disaffected housewives but as elders, 60 years old or older (Warren and Levy, 1991). Among patients of all ages there were men as well as women, including some Vietnam veterans and homeless males, and both male and female immigrants (Warren and Levy, 1991). As in the 1950s–1970s, some of the female ECT patients' case histories mixed psychiatric with social and reproductive role concerns and family relations, including postpartum psychosis, anorexia, menopause, obesity, pregnancy, and husbands seeking ECT for their wives. Among the medical records on petitions for involuntary ECT in the public defender's office of the Los Angeles Mental Health Court in the 1980s:

WF, age 32: husband brought to hospital, Russian born. Long standing stresses began a year ago when she married and they left Russia. Patient had not been away from her family. At first pleased with pregnancy, past 2–4 weeks started to become depressed . . . starving to death and in this manner endangers her unborn child.

WF, age 48: The patient has two children ages 4 and 9, she is a homemaker . . . the patient is dressed carelessly, looks her age. Husband wants her to have ECT because she had it in 1975 and it worked.

Korean F, age 24: She was depressed since birth of first of three children. She just gave birth to the third. Dr.'s letter says, "has been ill with depressive disorder psychotic features since 1985 after the birth of her children. She has done poorly since—and has been unable to return to her previous job."

Beginning as early as the mid-1970s, from available California data, ECT patients were middle to upper middle class, increasingly elderly as well as female and Anglo. In the decade between the mid-1970s and mid-1980s, the proportion of patients in California who were 60 years old or older rose from roughly one third to roughly one half (Warren and Levy, 1991). In the 1981 California Patients' Rights Office Report on ECT there were 2,451 patients treated with ECT; in 1990 the figure was 2,671, with 66 percent female, 47.7 percent 65 or older, and 89.6 percent Anglo (Mayer, 1991). By 1994 there were 2,356 patients, with 68.1 percent female, 50.6 percent 65 or older, and 90.1 percent Anglo (Kramer, 1999).

From a psychiatric perspective, this increase in the proportion of elderly among ECT patients was accounted for by the rise in depressive illness among the elderly population, together with tolerance for, and medical risks attendant upon, the use of psychopharmacology among elderly patients

(Gaspar and Samarasinghe, 1982; Lehmann, 1982; Pearlman, 1991). From a sociological perspective, changes in the U.S. social structure—including survival of proportionately more (and older) elderly together with more women at work and fewer caregivers in the home—also help to account for the increase in the proportion of elderly among ECT recipients (Warren and Levy, 1991).

Both sociologists and mental health practitioners concurred that was it was age more than gender issues that accounted for this proportional increase (Warren and Levy, 1991). Although there were more women than men among elderly ECT recipients during the 1980s–1990s, this is most likely because women survived, on average, longer than men. In terms of depressive illness, Lehmann claimed in 1982 that "the incidence and prevalence of depression are unduly high in the population over 60, more so among men than women" (p. 41). Just as some pro-ECT psychiatrists of the 1950s–1970s explained the greater proportion of women among ECT patients as a consequence of their greater liability to affective disorder, some practitioners of the 1980s–1990s made the same link between ECT, affective disorders, and old age.

Psychiatrists' case for the use of ECT among elderly depressed patients had three bases: the effect (or lack of it) of psychopharmaceuticals on elderly bodies, relative cost factors, and relative efficacy, especially with suicidal cases. Lehmann (1982: 41) noted the problem of psychoactive drugs' effect on "blood pressure, cardiac, and cognitive functions," while Pearlman (1991: 129) commented that ECT is useful with women in the third trimester of pregnancy and with elderly patients "because of possible complications of drugs." Pearlman also highlighted the cost of hospitalization in his comparison of ECT with psychopharmacology: "The significantly greater cost of hospitalization for patients who fail a drug trial before receiving ECT . . . raises questions about routine use of the most effective treatment last" (1991: 128).

But greater efficacy was the core of 1980s–1990s pro-ECT practitioners' arguments concerning the use of the treatment with elderly (and nonelderly) patients. Lehmann (1982: 39–40) called ECT "the most effective antidepressant treatment available," noting that to avoid memory deficits and confusion among elderly patients unilateral rather than bilateral ECT should be used, and the treatment should be limited to once or twice a week for a total of three to six treatments per course. Zimmer and Price (1991: 435) proposed that the use of ECT in geriatric depression should be "non-reckless but aggressive, thorough, and systematic." The resort to ECT was portrayed in the literature as a life-saving response to depression among elderly (and other) patients; one study of 45 ECT patients published in 1991 by Pearlman claimed that 16 of the consenting and 8 of the nonconsenting patients were in a "life threatening" psychiatric condition. Gaspar and Samarasinghe (1982), in England, said that half the "courses" of ECT given in their study of 33 patients aged 66–88 were given "because ECT was the only way of improving the patients. If antagonism to ECT were to increase through the efforts of the anti-ECT lobby, many elderly depressives would suffer much harm. For depressives who refuse to eat or drink, ECT is truly life saving" (p. 173). Practitioners who saw ECT as effective with suicidal patients proposed that its use not be limited to the "last resort," but, rather, it should be the first line of treatment (Pearlman, 1991). In addition to "first line," other concepts that reappeared in the pro-ECT literature during the 1980s–1990s included prophylactic ECT and maintenance ECT (Warren and Levy, 1991).

On both sides of the Atlantic, ECT practitioners used the treatment with elderly patients for a variety of diagnoses as well as depression, and cited impressive success rates, sometimes in comparison with other, and/or placebo treatments. Kellner and Bernstein (1993) described the use of ECT as a treatment for Parkinson's, strokes, dementia, neuroleptic malignant syndrome, catatonia, epilepsy, and delirium. Burke and his colleagues, in St. Louis (1985: 482), used ECT among elderly patients with major affective disorder (24), bipolar affective disorder (5), schizoaffective disorder (2), dementia (3), and somatization and dysthymic disorder (1). In Warren and Levy's (1991: 323) study of 41 involuntary ECT patients aged 60 or over, the diagnoses were similar: psychotic depression (18), depression (10), dementia/organic (8), bipolar (6), and schizophrenia (4).

Claimed improvement rates for ECT in clinical studies by practitioners hovered around 80 percent for elderly patients. In a chart review of 30 patients aged 60 or more in St. Louis, Burke and his colleagues noted that "twenty-five subjects (83 percent) improved with ECT. . . . Eighteen obtained complete remission and seven had partial resolution of their symptoms" (1985: 481). In New York, Meyers and Mei-Tal (1985) compared the outcomes of psychogeriatric treatment with psychopharmacology and ECT with 70 patients; relative effectiveness was greater with ECT (81.4 percent) than with psychopharmacy (62.5 percent). Mielke and his colleagues claimed that 18 of their MMECT (Multiple Monitored Electroconvulsive Therapy) patients over 60 had an excellent to good response, 5 moderate, 1 fair, and 1 poor (1984: 181).

Throughout the decades since the 1940s, both critics and practitioners of ECT have been concerned with the safety of shock machinery and procedures used; these concerns are, if anything, greater with respect to the frail elderly. As the reader might expect by now, anti-ECT psychiatrists and other critics were not impressed by the safety of "new" ECT machines and procedures, while ECT practitioners regarded the treatment as, overall, safe for both elderly and nonelderly patients—if they were "properly" diagnosed, medically worked-up, and handled during the treatment. Gaspar and Samarasinghe (1982: 173) reported few deaths and no complications among their 33 patients (with 384 ECT applications). Meyers and

Mei-Tal (1985: 120) complained that "It has been recognized that ECT is the safest and most effective treatment for the elderly with major depressive illness and is associated with a lower morbidity and mortality than other somatic therapies. . . . Nevertheless, TCA's were usually the initial modality of treatment on this unit." There were, however, some warnings in the literature: Burke and his colleagues (1985: 480) shared the general enthusiasm for elder ECT but noted that it should be used with caution, particularly among patients 75 or older with cardiovascular problems (see also Jefferson, 1983).

Some studies compared elderly with nonelderly patients' ECT outcomes. Alexopoulos and his colleagues (1984: 651) found in their New York chart study that 199 geriatric patients "developed significantly more medical problems that required medical treatment or temporary discontinuation of electroconvulsive therapy than did younger controls (N = 94). The most important of these were cardiovascular in nature." However, these authors, too, concluded that ECT was indicated in cases where the elder was anorexic or suicidal (p. 177).

Sociological studies focus on the social and cultural contexts of elderly ECT patienthood; the ways in which age-related expectations within the family can precipitate mental hospitalization and ECT. The proportion of people—especially women—surviving into old age increased steadily during the second half of the twentieth century. The traditional family caregivers of the 1950s—married women—were no longer in the home to care for children, let alone elderly parents. Elderly individuals living with mentally disordered husbands or wives, or adults taking care of their elderly parents, were liable to come to the end of their rope in caring for these individuals. Insurance, perhaps Medicare-funded psychiatric hospitalization (see below), formed one possible, if often temporary solution to such problems in caregiving. Once hospitalized, the "deviance" of the housewives of the 1950s was related to inadequately performed childcare and housework, and the husbands' to inadequately performed work roles (Warren, 1987). The out-of-role behavior of the 1980s elderly took the form of too much activity, or too little. Those who were inactive, vegetative or mute, refusing the self-care functions of toileting, feeding, or getting out of bed, were diagnosed with some form of depression, anorexia, or catatonia. Those who were overly active for the elderly—one patient had bought a red Corvette on credit—were diagnosed with mania or manic-depression (Warren and Levy, 1991). Once they were hospitalized, the likelihood of getting ECT was amplified by the existence of the machines in the hospital, the continuation of deviant behaviors on the ward, and a history of psychoactive drugs to which they had become tolerant (Warren and Levy, 1991). A typical case was that of an 80-year-old Anglo woman, who was admitted, at the behest of her husband, to a private hospital in Los Angeles: "Extremely agitated, paranoid, not eating or sleeping, not caring for personal hygiene, disheveled, anxious, confused, and can't care for self." She remained uncooperative with hospital personnel, "refused her medication, ignored hygiene" (*Public Defenders Office Records*, 1982)—and was scheduled for ECT.

Involuntary ECT was permitted for elderly (and nonelderly) patients in Los Angeles when they were judged, by the Mental Health Court, too incompetent to give or withhold consent (Warren and Levy, 1991). Their relatives tended, at first (having seen *One Flew Over the Cuckoo's Nest*) to be unwilling to permit the treatment, but were persuaded by hospital staff and by the videos that had been made to counteract *Cuckoo's Nest*'s imagery. A daughter said of her father's proposed ECT: "it seemed barbaric . . . no one could explain why it worked"; after the hospital's portrayal of the treatment as "legitimate and recognized" she gave her father's consent to the treatment. The daughter of a 77-year-old female patient said that she had seen *Cuckoo's Nest* and had "always equated ECT with that depiction"; however, she gave consent for her mother's treatment with ECT because, like another daughter of a 65-year-old woman, she was "at the end of my rope."

After the initial ECT—which might be the first in the elderly patient's life, or a renewal of the treatment after years or decades—relatives observed behavioral changes in the elders. The vegetative were more alert, the agitated calmer. Many of the relatives then became less hesitant about the treatment; one 50-year-old daughter, a clinical psychologist, stated that her prior "philosophical opposition" had changed to "endorsement," and she had even suggested it to some of her own patients. The elderly patients themselves were generally less sanguine about the effects of the treatment, hating the memory loss they experienced, and the stigma of mental hospitalization (Warren and Levy, 1991). Some feared death by ECT; others had lived long enough: "A 60-year-old man said, 'Don't let them give me ECT, I wouldn't survive it.' . . . When the public defender asked an 80-year-old woman why she was not eating and drinking and did not want the ECT, she replied, 'It's a little late' " (Warren and Levy, 1991: 319).

Researchers during the 1990s examined the other end of the age spectrum than elderly in relation to ECT use: children and adolescents. Baldwin and Oxlad (2000) published case histories and a "meta-analysis" of fifty years of electroshock with children in America and other countries. Their study indicates that (unlike adults) more boys than girls were given electroshock. The most recent (1994–1997) American ECT cases they cited included a 6-year-old boy with Tourette's syndrome, a girl diagnosed with posttraumatic stress disorder after a gang rape, and an African-American male who believed he had AIDS but was diagnosed with acute lymphocytic leukemia (Baldwin and Oxlad, 2000: 91, 116).

By the late 1990s, Texas and California were the only states that forbade the treatment of children under 12 with ECT. Reports of the treatment of children with ECT in the 1990s came from teaching hospitals such as UCLA (eight adolescents), the University Hospital of Stony Brook (thirteen patients ages 15–19), the University of Michigan (seven girls ages 14–17); and the

Mayo Clinic (ten girls and ten boys aged 18) (Logan, 1995). The conclusion of a Child Depression Consortium in the fall of 1994 was that ECT was indicated for adolescents diagnosed with "severe depressive states, mania, catatonia, and acute psychosis" and was "safe and . . . cost effective" for the young (Logan, 1995: 4). A 1994 study of ECT treatment of an 8-year-old girl diagnosed with catatonia said that she was problem free until "after her participation in a week-long summer camp; however, repeated questioning of several sources revealed no report of any unusual or traumatic event during her week at camp" (Cizadlo and Wheaton, 1995: 333). Judging the girl's treatment a success, Cizadlo and Wheaton reported several other cases of ECT treatment for "life-threatening catatonia in children: an 11-year-old boy, a 13-year-old boy, a 14-year-old girl, and an older adolescent" (1995: 332–333).

PATIENTS' VOICES: MEDIA PORTRAYALS AND CELEBRITY ENDORSEMENTS

During the 1980s–1990s, the tortured face of Jack Nicholson in *Cuckoo's Nest* was replaced in video imagery by the smiles of anonymous, newly awoken patients who had just been reborn through the pushbutton psychiatry of the new ECT. Although not all media treatments of ECT were positive (see, for example, Cauchon, 1995), many of them were. And quite a few celebrities lent their names and identities to the publicizing and endorsement of electroshock—the name itself even returning to psychiatric publication at the end of the century (Fink, 1999).

Even the patients' rights movement itself moved, during the 1990s, toward endorsement rather than criticism of ECT. The National Alliance for the Mentally Ill, an organization of patients and their families, urged that the treatment be made more accessible (Foderaro, 1993: A11). A growing number of experts in psychology who experienced ECT, from Norman Endler (1982) to Martha Manning (1995), advocated for the treatment during the last decades of the twentieth century, together with testimonials from celebrities such as novelist William Styron and actress Patty Duke Astin (Solomon, 1996: 20–22).

The shift in the public presentation of ECT from a form of torture to a miracle changed the metaphors from within which patients spoke of their experiences. In the 1960s and 1970s, patients spoke of sacrifice or crucifixion to describe their experiences with ECT (see Chapter 4); in the 1980s and 1990s, the language was one of resurrection and deliverance. As one ex-patient put it, "I actually start to love ECT. . . . It's like receiving a blessing in a sanctuary" (Behran, 1999: 67). Dick Cavett, recalling his experiences with ECT, said, "In my case, ECT was miraculous." When he first saw his wife after the treatment, he sat up in bed and said, "Look who's back among the living. It was like a magic wand" (Roan, 1992: 1). Producer Joshua Logan recalled that after his treatment, "All I wanted to do was lie there and enjoy this cool peace...flowing through me" (quoted in Rael and Armat, 1995: 156–157).

With the 1960s and 1970s critique of technology fading into history, the electrical power and machinery of ECT seemed for some (male) 1980s–1990s patients (as in the nineteenth century; see the Introduction and Chapter 2) the key to resurrection. A musician referred to his ECT treatment as a "Roto-Rooter" which "reamed me clear as the depression was gone" (Foderaro, 1993: 1). A mechanic in his 60s attributed the success of ECT to the power of the electrical: "There is something in your system that is not lined up anymore. That is not correct. . . . Because of all kinds of things that happened to me my brain waves were not any more corrected to the pattern. And the shock treatment had a great thing to do with that to get it back in shape again. Not so much the medication, because chemicals I don't like, but in electricity I believe. It makes cars go, it makes a household go, it makes everything go. It is part of our body system too" (Warren interview). One patient was so taken with ECT that denied maintenance treatments by his psychiatrist, he "treated" himself with periodic visits to an electrified cattle fence, to which he touched his forehead (Bishop, 1989: 1061).

The rebirth of ECT was not without opposition from patients and anti-ECT psychiatrists. After noting the media's fascination with the resurgence of ECT, Seth Farber appealed to "all individuals of conscience to step forward and oppose the resurgence of electroconvulsive therapy" (1991: 92). He also argued that the "new" ECT was not as different from the "old" as practitioners claimed (1991: 98). Legislative opposition to ECT came from the same general geopolitical areas that it had in previous decades; during 1991, the San Francisco Board of Supervisors voted to oppose the use and public financing of ECT (Farber, 1991: 2). But the words of patients praising electroshock at the *fin de siècle* overwhelmed the voices of opposition. Many of the themes in 1980s–1990s ECT can be seen in Martha Manning's 1994 memoirs, starting with her feeling, beginning in January 1990, that her life was out of control. Anxious and fearful, feeling inadequate and unable to experience pleasure, she sought psychiatric help, and was diagnosed with depression. After seven months of treatment with MAO (monoamine oxidase) inhibitors she showed no improvement, and her therapist recommended ECT, telling her that the treatment might be the last resort in the preservation of her sanity and even her life.

Manning's image of ECT was drawn from the film of *One Flew Over the Cuckoo's Nest*, and she imagined the electrical jolting of McMurphy and the Chief. The literature supplied by her doctor, in contrast, included the favorable 1985 NIMH consensus report on ECT. She read another study claiming that a majority of patients found ECT "no more distressing than a dental procedure" (1994: 101–102). She also learned of the economics of 1990s ECT: fees for the facility, anesthesiologist, nursing staff, and attending physician.

After her insurance company denied her benefits for outpatient ECT, Manning entered the clinic at a local hospital as an inpatient (1994: 110–117). Briefed by her physicians the night before her treatment, she wrote, "Tomorrow morning I will be awakened at 5 A.M. for a shot of atropine, used to dry secretions" (1994: 120). Once in the ECT room she would be "attached to monitors that will register the activity of my heart and my brain. A band will be fastened around my head . . . several electrodes will be placed over the temporal region of my non-dominant hemisphere." She would be given oxygen through a mask, while an IV supplied both an anaesthetic and a muscle relaxant to prevent "the breakage of bones." Once prepared, she would receive "between 80 and 170 volts" causing "a *grand mal* seizure that will last for between thirty and sixty-five seconds"; after 15 to 30 minutes, she would awaken (1994: 120–121).

Martha Manning had six ECT treatments between October 17 and 31. She remembered these treatments much as Sylvia Plath did a half century earlier, as erotic, religious, infused with female passivity and practitioner dominance; she described "offering myself up to these strangers in exchange for the possibility of deliverance. Someone holds my hands and slips needles under my skin. Another slides down my gown and plants red valentine hearts on my chest. Fingers anoint my temples with cool ointment and fasten a plastic crown tightly around my head" (1994: 124). Unlike Plath's, Manning's memories were of kindliness, and the perceived outcome of her treatment a success: "I remember the gentleness of the voices and hands, so different from the violence I expected. . . . I remember my doctor whispering softly, 'Go to sleep now . . .' " (1995: 171). Later she recalled sitting in her car watching "as my daughter emerges from the cluster of kids pouring out of the school door. Old joys are resurrected in my heart. My mouth and eyes remember how to smile. I appreciate the perfection of a moment" (1995: 171).

As the prototypical patient of the late twentieth century, Martha Manning was female, well educated, middle class, and white. She had been brought to ECT after discovering that for her, as for many other patients, drugs were not the "magic bullet" they had seemed a decade or so earlier. The physicians who led her to ECT were careful—unlike those of the 1950s and 1960s (Warren, 1987)—about informed consent, providing her with technical details of the ECT treatment she would receive. She submitted to the treatment as the woman on the couch did in the nineteenth century, and Sylvia Plath 40 years earlier, lying down at the behest of the doctor. The key to the economics of the treatment was her insurance company, which denied outpatient but permitted inpatient ECT. The major difference between Manning and the most typical 1990s mental patient was her age: she was not over 60.

By 1999, in the words of Max Fink, "The indications for ECT have been broadened . . . it has gone from being a last resort for unresponsive depressed and suicidal patients to being a treatment option for patients with delusional

pression, mania, schizophrenia . . . catatonia . . . parkinsonism and . . .
uroleptic drug toxicity" (pp. 106–107). This rebirth of electroshock therapy
ntinued into the twenty-first century, bracketed by both theold—Western,
triarchal gendered electrotherapeutics—and the "new"—American tech-
logies, economics, and legalities. Videos, computer-assisted ECT machines,
d corporation-psychiatrist ties may be new, but the hierarchies of class and
nder in psychiatric diagnosis and treatment, the fusion of medical with
ltural imagery and language, are not. In the first decade of the twenty-first
ntury, electroshock appears, as we shall see in the Epilogue, in other places,
th old and new. Together with magnetism, electrical treatment is part of the
rival of folk medicine we call "New Age." And it appears, as do all things
emingly, in the new world of the World Wide Web.

Epilogue
Into the Twenty-First Century

In the first decade of the twenty-first century electroconvulsive therapy remained at the forefront of electrical treatments for mental illness, spearheaded by pro-ECT psychiatrists such as Richard Abrams and Max Fink. In 1992, Abrams wrote that "Only four years have elapsed since the first edition [1988] of this volume, hardly enough time, it would seem, for the ink to dry, yet the present edition is over 100 pages longer and contains more than 350 new references…..For the sixth straight decade, clinical advances in ECT have outstripped an understanding of their mechanisms, leaving society in possession of a highly effective and essentially risk-free method of relieving melancholia and other mental disorder" (p. vii-viii). Fink, who is at work on his own history of electroshock, has also promoted the financial savings when ECT rather than tricyclic antidepressants are used in inpatient care, and laments that too "few managed care insurers recognize the merits of ECT, either as a relief for their insured ill patients or as a financial benefit to their shareholders" (1999: p. 109).

Indeed, the case for ECT has been made successfully at least in California, where statistics are mandated from both the public and the private sector (see Ch. 5). The number of patients of ECT in California almost doubled between 1994 and 2004, from 2,356 patients to 4,553 patients. Two thirds of the ECT treatments in California were given to women and 81.7% to white nonminorities, statistics that did not change much during the decade. The percentage of treatments given to persons 65 and older declined from over a half to just under a third, with the 45-64 age group the most likely to receive ECT at just over a third of the total (Office of Human Rights, 2004).

ECT continued to engender controversy between those psychiatrists, patients and others who endorsed the treatment, and those psychiatrists, patients and others who opposed it. A pro-ECT website, www.electroshock. org (2000) provided links to ECT physicians, clinical studies, and Dr. Fink's 1999 book. An anti-ECT website, www.ect.org (2008) featured patient horror stories, a "hall of shame" directed at ECT practitioners, and a discussion of the website licensee's ties to the pharmaceutical company.

The popularity of alternate forms of electrotherapy is also on the rise, mirroring events at the turn of the last century. Other forms of electrotherapy being used in the first decade of the twenty-first century for the treatment of depression and other mental conditions include electric light treatment, hich in the nineteenth century was called "photochromatic treatment" ritchard-Davies, 1877).   Electric light treatment is proposed—with oogle checkout—as a treatment for SAD: Seasonal Affective Disorder or asonal Affective Depression. One of many "phototherapy" internet sites 2008 sold BlueMax lamps costing around $150 each. This site featured stimonials from users, apparently using their own names, reminiscent of lvertisements found as early as the eighteenth century:

> I had SAD and my grandson was depressed and after sitting with the UltraLux 11 and desk lamp we are new people! (www.fullspectrumsolutions.com)

Pritchard-Davies (1877:344) in the nineteenth century also claimed at his "nervous" patients were helped by the light in the "blue room," though not by the light in the "red room."

Cranial Electric Stimulation, which originated in the early twentieth ntury as electrosleep (see the Introduction), gained momentum in the 2000s an alternative to drugs and electroshock in the treatment of depression ilula and Kirsch, 2005). CES machines, sold by eight companies over the ternet, were advertised as a cost-effective alternative to the pharmaceutical eatment of depression, anxiety, or insomnia. As Class 11a Type B devices, ES machines had "clip-on electrodes attached to the earlobes" (Gilula and rsch, 2005: 11) and were sold to physicians, who could then sell them to order them for patients. CES patients themselves administer electrical imulation to their brains. The website of a company selling "Alpha-Stim" ES machines also featured testimonials from users, again apparently ing their own names. One 60 year old woman reported that she had been pressed since the age of 5 and had tried antidepressants to no avail. After e ordered and used the Alpha-Stim machine she experienced

> an immediate lifting of the 'cloud'....After 7 months of daily use I have experienced no side effects and am completely off antidepressant drugs. (www. alphastim.com 2008).

Magnetism, too, continued its centuries-long debate with the electrical. ans-Cranial Magnetic Stimulation (TMS) refers to the stimulation of the rebral cortex with low frequency (once per second) or high frequency (>5 r second) magnetic pulses. Low frequency TMS, used in the treatment auditory hallucinations, is said to decrease brain activity, while high- equency TMS, used in the treatment of depression, is said to increase (www.neuronetics.com 2008). By 2008, around 1500 patients had been ated with TMS, which is administered by a physician. There were several mpanies making TMS machines, all claiming that the treatment is more ccessful than alternative electrical or pharmaceutical approaches.

On their respective websites, TMS and ECT purveyors made claims, in the st decade of the twenty-first century, for the greater value of their products in e treatment of depression and other mental illnesses. Neuronetics, maker of

ie Neurostar TMS machine, claimed that "A principal benefit of TMS is that
requires no electrical connection to the body as required for ECT"(www.
euronetics.com 2007); Somatics LLC, maker of the ECT machine Thymatron—
eferring to low-frequency TMS as a nonconvulsive and high-frequency TMS
s a convulsive treatment (www.thymatron.com 2008)—said that:

> Nonconvulsive TMS … is likely to be a useful addition to available treatment
> choices for depression; however, it seems unlikely that it will ever replace ECT
> in the more severe (e.g. melancholic) forms of depression…[there is] little chance
> that [convulsive TMS] could exhibit greater therapeutic potency than ECT.

TMS proponents counterclaimed that "Magnetic stimulation may be as
ffective as ECT in treating severe depression." (www.anxiety-depression-
lternatives.com (2008)

CES, TMS, and ECT are used and sold as treatment options in
nainstream medicine. Various other iterations of alternative, folk or quack
lectrical and magnetic medicine are advertised and sold at the intersection
f the "New Age" with profitmaking. Magnetic bracelets and rings, sold
hrough the internet or mail order, promise relief from arthritis or stress.
amber "can be worn or used by people that…get depressed easily" (www.
nikalina.com 2008), or for anxiety; it "carries a negative electrical energy
harge and therefore is good to draw power and energy into its bearer"
www.shgresources.com 2008)—paid for by your gold credit card.

Variations of animal, as well as mineral, magnetism could be found
n the cornucopia of early twentieth century treatments, echoing the
healing at a distance" of ancient, premodern and modern times. Clinical
iypnotism or hypnotherapy, was "more and more popular" in the
reatment of alcoholism and smoking disorders (www.hypnosecrets.com
008), drawing upon the unseen powers that move between patient and
realer. At the borderland of mainstream medicine, Therapeutic Touch—
irst developed in the 1970s— was provided by members of the Nurse
Iealers Professional Associates International (www.therapeutictouch.
rg 2008). Therapeutic Touch does not actually involve touch; instead,
he nurse practitioner holds "the hands 2 to 6 inches away from the
ndividual's energy field while moving the hands from the head to the
eet in a rhythmical, symmetrical manner."

ECT and other electrical treatments for mental disorders are an
ntegral part of both American culture and the cultural history of the
Vest. America's fascination with technology and marketing are reflected
n the ways in which electrotherapy developed here during the last four
enturies. But the medical traditions within which American technology
nd marketing developed partake of ancient themes in Western culture:
rgans and fluids; body and mind; balance and moderation; electricity and
nagnetism. We seem, in the twenty-first century, to be where we began, in
world in which healing can be at a distance or tethered to a machine.

Epilogue

And so, this is the end of our cultural history of pushbutton psychiatry; a tale of Europe as well as America; of change and continuity in technology, disciplinary power and economics; of gender, power and knowledge hierarchies. A tale of ECT to be sure, but also one of medicine in Western culture, with its cycles of (re)invention, immersion, institutionalization, backlash, retrenchment—(re)invention. Ours is one interpretation of the ways in which the human body and the natural world intertwine with culture and technology in history. Turning our gaze upon ECT is one of the myriad ways in which we can learn to see not only our society, but also ourselves in a mirror; what we make, at any given moment in time and space, of our bodies, minds and madness.

Bibliography

ARCHIVAL SOURCES

Blain, Daniel. Papers. American Psychiatric Association Archives, Washington, D.C.
Joint Information Services Files. American Psychiatric Association Archives, Washington, D.C.
Public Defenders Office Records. Mental Health Court, Los Angeles, California.

PUBLISHED SOURCES

Titles

American Journal of Psychiatry (1941), 98.
American Journal of Psychiatry (1943), 100.
American Journal of Psychiatry (1958), 115.
Annual Meeting (1870). *American Journal of Insanity* 27:157, 464–498.
A Comeback for Shock Therapy? (1979). *Time*, 19 November, 76.
Convulsive Therapy Bulletin with Tardive Dsykenesia Notes (1975), p. 172.
Brain Galvanizing Machine (1910). Flyer/Advertisement. Minneapolis: Bakken Library.
Dr. George Beard on Insanity (1880). *American Journal of Insanity* 37:229–236.
Depression and Electroshock (1972). *Newsweek*, 7 August, 20.
Diseases of the Nervous System (1955), 1, August.
ECT Use in Massachusetts: Found Down After State Regulation (1984). *Psychiatric News*, 16 April, 12.
ect.org. (1999). Available online at http://ect.org.
Electric Shock Findings (1949). *Newsweek*, 33, 17 January, 43.
Electric Shock Causes Partial Memory Loss (1940). *Science News Letter* 38, 20 September, 385.
electroshock.org. (1999). Available online at http://electroshock.org.
Fits Produced As Protection Against Epileptic Seizures (1941). *Science News Letter* 39, 21 June, 387.
Giant Power Heidelberg Electric Belt (1901). Sears catalog. Minneapolis: Bakken Library.
Insanity Treated by Electric Shock (1940). *New York Times*, 6 July, 17.
Latest News on Shock Treatments (1947). *Science Digest* 22, August, 30–31.
Mentally Ill Now Getting Shock Treatments (1942). *Science News Letter* 41, 30 May, 345.
New Horizons in Psychiatry (1948). *New York Times*, 3 January, 12.
New Society (1975). *Psychiatric News*, 19 November, 1.
Obituary (1917). Arthur Clapp. *American Journal of Electrotherapuetics and Radiology* 34:576.
Problem a Closed Chapter, Eagelton Candid (1972). *Chicago Tribune*, 26 July, 4.

Reclassification of ECT Devices Delayed (1984). *Psychiatric News*, 6 April, 143.
Reports for Hospitals of the Insane, 1869 (1870). *American Journal of Insanity*, 338.
Shock Affects Memory (1945). *Science News Letter* 49:230.
Shock for Mental Illness (1949). *Science News Letter* 55:139.
Shock Therapy: What it Means (1972). *Chicago Tribune*, 26 July, 4.
World Almanac (1915). New York: Press Publishing.
Zoist, the Journal of Cerebral Physiology and Mesmerism and Their Application to Human Welfare (1848–1849). London: Hyppolyte Ballière.

Authors

Abrams, R. (1989). Out of the Blue: The Rehabilitation of Electroconvulsive Therapy. *The Sciences* 29:24–28.
———. (1990). *Electroconvulsive Therapy*. 2nd ed. Oxford: Oxford University Press.
Accornero, F. (1988). An Eyewitness Account of the Discovery of Electroshock. *Convulsive Therapy* 4:41–49.
Adair, N., & Adair, C. (1978). *Word Is Out: Stories of Some of Our Lives*. San Francisco: New Glide Publications.
Adams, G.W. (1952). *Doctors in Blue: The Medical History of the Union Army*. New York: H. Schuman.
Adams, H. (1918). *The Education of Henry Adams*. Boston: Houghton Mifflin.
Adamson, G. (1955). Electroshock. *The Manitoba Medical Review* 35:14.
Adas, M. (1989). *Machines As the Measure of Men: Science, Technologies and Ideologies of Western Dominance*. Ithaca: Cornell University Press.
Aden, G. (1977). Effects of Restrictive Legislation of Electroconvulsive Therapy at a Freestanding Psychiatric Hospital. *Diseases of the Nervous System* 38:230–233.
———. (1984a). From the Desk of the Visiting Editor. *American Journal of Social Psychiatry* 4 (fall):6–8.
———. (1984b). The International Psychiatric Association for the Advancement of Electrotherapy: A Brief History. *American Journal of Social Psychiatry* 4 (fall):9–10.
———. (1984c). The Status of ECT As Therapeutic Modality in 1979. *American Journal of Social Psychiatry* 4 (fall):18–21.
Aldini, G. (1803). *An Account of the Late Improvements in Galvanism*. London: Cuticle and Martin.
Aldrich, C.K. (1955). *Psychiatry for the Family Practice*. New York: McGraw Hill.
Alexander, F.G., & Selesnick, S. (1966). *The History of Psychiatry: An Evaluation of Psychiatric Thought and Practice from Prehistoric Times to the Present*. New York: Harper and Row.
Alexander, L. (1953). *Treatment of Mental Disorders*. Philadelphia: W.B. Sanders.
Alexopoulos, G.S., Shamoian, C.J., Lucas, J., Weiser N., & Berger, H. (1984). Medical Problems of Geriatric Psychiatric Patients and Younger Controls During Electroconvulsive Therapy. *Journal of the American Geriatric Society* 32:651–654.
Allbutt, C.T. (1884). *Visceral Neuroses*. London: Churchill.
Alper, T.G. (1948). An Electric Shock Patient Tells His Story. *The Journal of Abnormal and Social Psychology* 43:201–210.

Alpers, B., & Hughes, J. (1942a). Brain Changes in Electrically Induced Convulsions in Humans. *Journal of Neuropathology and Experimental Neurology* 1:385–398.

––––. (1942b). Changes in the Brain After Electrically Induced Convulsions in Cats. *Archives of Neurology and Psychiatry* 47:385.

Althuis, J. (1860). *A Treatise on Medical Electricity: Theoretical and Practical*. Philadelphia: Lindsay and Blakiston.

Alverno, L. (1990). The Origins of Electroconvulsive Therapy. *Wisconsin Medical Journal* 89:54–56.

Amberson, W.R. (1958). The Influence of Fashion in the Development of Knowledge Concerning Electricity and Magnetism. *American Scientist* 46:33–50.

American Psychiatric Association. (1944). *One Hundred Years of American Psychiatry, 1844–1944*. New York: Columbia University Press.

––––. (1978). *Electroconvulsive Therapy: Report of the Task Force of the American Psychiatric Association*. Washington, D.C.: American Psychiatric Association.

––––. (1980). *Diagnostic and Statistical Manual of Mental Disorders*. 3rd ed. Washington, D.C.: American Psychiatric Association.

––––. (1985). ECT: New Study in How, Why, Who. *APA Monitor*, March, 18–19.

––––. (1994). *Diagnostic and Statistical Manual of Mental Disorders*. 4th ed. Washington, D.C.: American Psychiatric Association.

Andreasen, N. (1984). *The Broken Brain: The Biological Revolution in Psychiatry*. New York: Harper and Row.

Applebaum, P. (1994). *Almost a Revolution: Mental Health and the Limits to Change*. New York: Oxford University Press.

Arieti, S., ed. (1959). *American Handbook of Psychiatry*. Vol. 2. New York: Basic Books.

Armstrong, J. (1837). *Lectures on the Morbid Anatomy, Nature, and Treatment of Acute and Chronic Diseases*. Philadelphia: Desilver, Thomas, and Co.

Armstrong, T. (1991). The Electrification of the Body at the Turn of the Century. *Textual Practice* 5:303–325.

Ashwell, S. (1848). *A Practical Treatise on the Diseases Peculiar to Women*. Philadelphia: Lea and Blanchard.

Asnis, G.M., Fink, M., & Saferstein, S. (1978). ECT in Metropolitan New York Hospitals: A Survey of Practice. *American Journal of Psychiatry* 135:479–482.

Aspiz, H. (1987). Sexuality and the Pseudo-Sciences. In *Pseudo-Sciences and Society in the Nineteenth Century*, ed. Arthur Wrobel. Kentucky: University Press of Kentucky.

Augustin, F.L. (1803). *Versuch Einer Vollanstandigen Systematischen Geschichte der Galvanischen Electricitat Und Ihrer Medicinischen Anwendung*. Berlin: Felischeschen Buchandlung.

Babigian, H.M., & Guttmacher, L.B. (1984). Epidemiological Consideration in Electroconvulsive Therapy. *Archives of General Psychiatry* 41:246–253.

Badger, R. (1979). *The Great American Fair*. Chicago: Nelson Hall.

Bailine, S.H. (1998). Reimbursement and Documentation in an Ambulatory ECT Program. *Journal of ECT* 14:255–258.

Bailine, S.H., & Rau, J.H. (1981). The Decision to Use ECT: A Retrospective Study. *Comprehensive Psychiatry* 22:274–281.

Baker, A.B., ed. (1955). *Clinical Neurology*. New York: Hoeber Harper.

Baldwin, N. (1995). *Edison Inventing the Century*. New York: Basic Books.

Baldwin, S., & Oxlad, M. (2000). *Electroshock and Minors: A Fifty-Year Review.* Westport, CT: Greenwood Press.

Bale, H. (1951). Modern Treatment of Mental Illness Helps Many to Recover at East Moline Hospital. *Rock Island Argus,* 4 May, 12.

Banay, R.S. (1953). Preferred Approach to Paranoid States With Prolonged Non-Convulsive Electro-Shock Stimulation. *Confina Neurologia* 13:354–362.

Banzak, D. (1996). ECT: A Guide for Family Physicians. *American Family Physician* 53:273–281.

Barker, G.F. (1880). Some Modern Aspects of the Life Question. *Science* 1:112–118.

Barrera, S.E., Lewis, N.D.C., Pacella, B., & Kalinowsky, L. (1942). Brain Changes Associated with Electrically Induced Seizures. *Transactions of the American Neurological Association* 68:31–35.

Bartholow, R. (1890). Present Status of Electrotherapeutics. *Journal of Electrotherapeutics* 8:169–174.

Barton, W. (1987). *The History and Influence of the American Psychiatric Association.* Washington, D.C.: American Psychiatric Association.

Batz, J. (1996). A Kinder Gentler Shock. *The Riverfront Times,* 21 October, 9–15.

Beard, G. (1869). Neurasthenia (Nervous Exhaustion). *Boston Medical and Surgical Journal* 80:217–221.

———. (1873–1874). The Treatment of Insanity by Electricity. *Journal of Mental Science* 19:355.

———. (1874a). Cases of Hysteria, Neurasthenia, Spinal Irritation and Allied Affections with Remarks. *Journal of Nervous and Mental Diseases,* 438–451.

———. (1874b). Miscellaneous Notes. *Archives of Electrology and Neurology* 1:438–451.

———. (1881). *American Nervousness: Its Causes and Consequences.* New York: G. Putnam's Sons.

———. (1972). *Sexual Neurasthenia.* New York: Arno Press, 1898. Reprint *New York Times.*

Beard, G., & Rockwell, A.D. (1867). *A Practical Treatise on the Medical and Surgical Uses of Electricity.* New York: William Wood.

———. (1881). *A Practical Treatise on the Medical and Surgical Uses of Electricity.* 3rd ed. New York: William Wood.

Beck, C., & Shennan, S. (1991). *Amber in Prehistoric Britain.* Oxford: Oxbow Books.

Becker, H. (1961). *Social Thought from Lore to Science.* 3rd ed. New York: Dover.

Becker, H.S. (1963). *Outsiders: Studies in the Sociology of Deviance.* New York: Free Press.

Behran, A. (1999). Electroboy. *New York Times Magazine,* 17 January, 67.

Bell, L. (1980). *Treating the Mentally Ill from Colonial Times to the Present.* New York: Praeger.

Bender, L. (1947). One Hundred Cases of Childhood Schizophrenia Treated with Electric Shock. *Transactions of the American Neurological Society* 72:165–196.

Benjamin, P. (1989). *A History of Electricity: The Intellectual Rise in Electricity.* New York: John Wiley.

Bennett, H.C. (1912). *The Electrotherapeutic Guide or a Thousand Questions Asked and Answered.* 9th ed. Lima, Ohio: National College of Electrotherapeutics.

Bernucci, R., & Glass, A., eds. (1973). *Neuropsychiatry in World War II.* Vol. II, *Overseas Theater.* Washington, D.C.: Office of Surgeon General.

Berrios, G.E. (1997). The Scientific Origins of Electroconvulsive Therapy: A Conceptual History. *History of Psychiatry* 8:105–119.

Beveridge, A.W., & Renvoize, E.B. (1988). Electricity: A History of its Use in the Treatment of Mental Illness in Britain During the Second Half of the Nineteenth Century. *British Journal of Psychiatry* 153:157–162.

Birch, J. (1799). Letter on Medical Electricity. In George Adams, *An Essay on Electricity*. 5th ed. London: J. Dillon.

———. (1800). *Consideration of the Efficacy of Electricity in Removing Female Obstructions*. 2nd ed. London: T. Cadell.

Bird, G. (1860). *Lectures on Electricity and Galvanism*. Philadelphia: W.H. Hazard.

Bishop, F.B. (1899). Address of the President. *Transactions of the Annual Meeting of the American Electrotherapeutic Society* 9:16–22.

Bishop, L.C. (1989). Attempted Self-Administration of Electroconvulsive Therapy. *Southern Medical Journal* 82:1061–1062.

Blustein, B.E. (1979). New York Neurologists and the Specialization of American Medicine. *Bulletin of the History of Medicine* 53:170–183.

———. (1981). A Hollow Square of Psychological Science: American Neurologists and Psychiatrists in Conflict. In *Madhouses, Mad-doctors, and Madmen: The Social History of Psychiatry in the Victorian Era*, ed. Andrew Scull. Philadelphia: University of Pennsylvania Press.

Bockoven, J.S. (1956). Moral Treatment in American Psychiatry. *Journal of Nervous and Mental Disease* 124:167–194.

Bockris, V. (1994). *Transformer: The Lou Reed Story*. New York: Simon & Schuster.

Boodman, S. (1996). Shock Therapy: It's Back. *Washington Post*, 24 September, 14.

Boswell, J. (1993). Scientologists Pleased with ECT Legislation. *Texas Medicine* 89:7–8.

Bower, B. (1985). Panel Okays ECT, Calls for U.S. Survey. *Science News* 127 (22 July):389.

Boyce, C.W. (1880). *Electricity*. Chicago: W.A. Chatterton.

Bozarth, O.M. (1976). Shock: The Gentleman's Way to Beat Up a Woman. *Madness Network News* (June):27.

Braceland, F. (1947). Psychiatric Lessons from World War II. *American Journal of Psychiatry* 103:587–593.

Bracket, C.F. et al. (1890). *Electricity in Daily Life: A Popular Account of the Applications of Electricity in Everyday Uses*. New York: Charles Scribner's Sons.

Bradford, R.W., & Peacock, T.G. (1955). *One Hundred Thirteenth Annual Report of Milledgeville State Hospital*, 24–25.

Braslow, J. (1997). *Mental Ills and Bodily Cures*. Berkeley: University of California Press.

Breggin, P. (1979). *Electroshock: Its Brain Disabling Effects*. New York: Springer.

———. (1991). *Toxic Psychiatry: Why Therapy, Empathy, and Love Must Replace the Drugs, Electroshock, and Biochemical Theories of the New Psychiatry*. New York: St. Martin's Press.

Brill, H., & Patton R. (1957). Analysis of 1955–1956 Population Fall in New York State Mental Hospitals in First Year of Large Scale Use of Tranquilizing Drugs. *American Journal of Psychiatry* 114:509–517.

Briska, W. (1997). *The History of the Elgin Mental Health Center*. Carpentersville, IL: Crossroads.

Britten, E.H. (1875). *The Electric Physician*. Boston: William Britten.

Bromberg, W. (1982). *Psychiatry Between the Wars, 1918–1945. A Recollection*. Westport, CT: Greenwood Press.

Brown, T. (1817). *The Ethereal Physician*. Albany, NY: G.J. Loomis and Co.

Bubier, E.T. (n.d.). *Electrotherapeutic Handbook*. New York: Manhattan Electrical Supply Co.

Buck, A.H., ed. (1885). *A Reference Handbook of the Medical Sciences by Various Writers*. Vol. 1. New York: William Wood.

Bunker, A. (1944). American Psychiatric Literature During the Last One Hundred Years. In *One Hundred Years of American Psychiatry*. New York: Columbia University Press.

Bunnel, P. (1873). *Catalogue and Price List*. Philadelphia: Rue and Jones.

Burke, W.J., Rutherford, J.L, Zorumski, C.F., & Reich, T. (1985). Electroconvulsive Therapy and the Elderly. *Comprehensive Psychiatry* 26:480–486.

Burnham, J.C. (1967). Psychoanalysis and American Medicine: 1894–1918. *Psychological Issues* 5.

Butler State Hospital. (1953). *Annual Report for the Year 1953*.

Cadwallader-Evans, Mr. (1754). A Relation of a Cure Performed by Electricity. *Medical Observations and Inquiries* 1, 21 October.

Callan, J.P. (1979). Electroconvulsive Therapy. *Journal of the American Medical Association* 242:545–546.

Cameron, D. (1994). ECT: Sham Statistics, the Myth of Convulsive Therapy and the Case for Consumer Misinformation. *The Journal of Mind and Behavior* 15 (winter and spring):177–198.

Carpenter, Lewis G., Jr. (1953). An Experimental Test of an Hypothesis for Predicting Outcome with Electroshock Therapy. *The Journal of Psychology* 36:131–135.

Carpue, J.C. (1803). *An Introduction to Electricity and Galvanism*. London: A. Phillips, Longman and Rees, Cadell and Davies.

Cash, P., & Hoekstra, C.S. (1941). Use of Preliminary Curarization with Electroshock Therapies. *Archives of Neurology and Psychiatry* 45:857–860.

Cauchon, D. (1995). Electroshock: Controversy and Questions. *USA Today*, 6–7 December, 6D, 4D.

Cavallo, T. (1780). *An Essay on the Theory and Practice of Medical Electricity*. London: T. Cavallo.

Central State Hospital. (1943). *Ninety-Fifth Annual Report*. Indianapolis: C.E. Pauley and Co.

Cerletti, U. (1938). A New Method of Shock Therapy: "Electroconvulsive Treatment." In *The Origins of Modern Psychiatry*, ed. C. Thompson. London: John Wiley & Sons.

———. (1950). Old and New Information About Electroshock. *American Journal of Psychiatry* 107:87–94.

———. (1954). Electroshock Therapy. *Journal of Clinical and Experimental Psychopathology and Quarterly Review of Psychiatry and Neurology* 15:191–217.

Champion, T.D. (1984). *Prehistoric Europe*. London: Academic Press.

Channing, W.F. (1849). *Notes on the Medical Application of Electricity*. Boston: Davis Daniel, Jr.

Chant, C. (1989). *Science, Technology and Everyday Life, 1870–1950*. New York: Routledge.

Cizaldo, B.C., & Wheaton, A. (1995). Case Study: ECT Treatment of a Young Girl with Catatonia. *Journal of the American Academy of Child and Adolescent Psychiatry* 34:332–335.

Clapp, G.M. (1899). Electrotherapeutics a Science? *Journal of Electrotherapeutics* 17:13–21.

Clark, E., & Jacyna, L.S. (1987). *Nineteenth-Century Origins of Neuroscientific Concepts.* Berkeley: University of California Press.

Clark, M., & Lubenow, G.C. (1975). Attack on Electroshock. *Newsweek,* 17 March, 86.

Clark, M., Schmidt, M., & Hager, M. (1982). Voting on Electroshock. *Newsweek,* 25 October, 105.

Cleaves, M. (1910). *The Autobiography of a Neurasthene.* Boston: Gorham Press.

Closson, J.H., & Swaney, C. (1941). Electric Shock Therapy, Preliminary Report. *Archives of Neurology and Psychiatry* 46:943–946.

Cohen, I.B. (1990). *Benjamin Franklin's Science.* Cambridge: Harvard University Press.

Colwell, H.A. (1992). *An Essay on the History of Electrotherapy and Diagnosis.* London: William Heinmann.

Committee for the Truth in Psychiatry. What You Should Know About ECT, Available online at http://www.harborside.com/home/e/equinox/ect.htm (accessed August 29, 2001).

Coombe, A. (1834). *Observations on Mental Derangement.* Boston: Marsh, Capen and Lyon. Facsimile ed., Scholars' Facsimiles and Reprints, Delmar, New York, 1972.

Copp, O. (1921). Some Problems Confronting the Association. *American Journal of Psychiatry* 78 (July):1–13.

Cornwall, P. (1991). *Body of Evidence.* New York: Avon Books.

Cotton, H. (1930). The Role of Physiotherapy in the Treatment of Mental Disorders. *Physical Therapeutics* 48:57–68.

Cushing, P. (1995). *Constructing the Self, Constructing America: A Cultural History of Psychotherapy.* Reading, MA: Addison-Wesley.

Dain, N. (1989). Critics and Dissenters: Reflections on "Anti-Psychiatry" in the United States. *Journal of the History of the Behavioral Sciences* 25:2–12.

———. (1994). Anti-Psychiatry in the United States. In *Discovering the History of Psychiatry,* ed. Mark Micale and Roy Porter. New York: Oxford.

Dana, C.L. (1904). The Partial Passing of Neurasthenia. *Journal of Nervous and Mental Disease* 31:191–193.

———. (1928). Early Neurology in the United States. *Journal of the American Medical Association* 90 (5 May):1421–1425.

———. (1925). *Textbook of Nervous Diseases.* 10th ed. New York: William Wood.

Darnton, R. (1968). *Mesmerism and the End of the Enlightenment in France.* Cambridge: Harvard University Press.

DeKraft, F. (1916). Report of the Committee on High Frequency Current. *American Journal of Electrotherapeutics and Radiology* 34:5–13.

Delaware State Hospital. (1941). *Twenty-Sixth Biennial Report.* Wilmington, DE: Star Publishing.

Dent, E.D. (1903). Hydrotherapy More Systematic. *American Journal of Insanity* 59:91.

Deutsch, A. (1948). *Shame of the States.* New York: Harcourt Brace.

———. (1949). *The Mentally Ill in America. A History of Their Care and Treatment from Colonial Times.* 2nd ed. New York: Columbia University Press.

Dewees, W.P. (1828). *Treatise on the Diseases of Females.* 2nd ed. Philadelphia: Carey, Lea and Carey.

Diefendorf, A.R. (1923). *Clinical Psychiatry.* New York: Macmillan Co.

Dowboggin, I. (1991). *Inheriting Madness.* Berkeley: University of California Press.

Drobes, S. (1946). Present Status of Electroshock Therapy. *Connecticut Medical Journal* 10:903–907.

Duck, J.J. (1912). *Anything Electrical.* Toledo, OH: n.p.

Dugan, W.J. (1910). *Handbook of Electrotherapeutics.* Philadelphia: F.A. Davis.

Dunham, H.W., & Weinberg, S.K. (1960). *The Culture of the State Mental Hospital.* Detroit: Wayne State University Press.

Dwyer, E. (1987). *Homes for the Mad: Life Inside Two Nineteenth-Century Asylums.* New Brunswick, NJ: Rutgers University Press.

Earle, P. (1877). Curability of Insanity. *American Journal of Insanity* 33:483–533.

East Moline State Hospital. (1940–1941). *Annual Report East Moline State Hospital.* East Moline, IL.

———. (1963). *Annual Report East Moline State Hospital.* East Moline, IL.

Eastern State Hospital. (1999). Available online at http://www.easternstatehospital.org.

Eastgate, J. (1998). The Case Against Electroshock. *USA Today Weekend.* 12 November, 28.

Ebaugh, F.G., Barnacle, C.H., & Neubeurger, K.T. (1943). Fatalities Following Electric Convulsive Therapy. *Archives of Neurology and Psychiatry* 49:107–117.

Eberhart, N.M. (1913). *A Brief Guide to Vibratory Technique.* 3rd ed. Chicago: New Medicine Publishing Co.

Eberle, J. (1842). *A Treatise of the Materia Medica and Therapeutics.* Philadelphia: Griggs and Eliott.

Edison, T. (1948). Thomas Edison on Life Units. In *The Diary and Sundry Observations of Thomas Alva Edison.* New York: Philosophical Library.

———. (1991). *The Papers of Thomas Edison.* Vol. 2, *From Workshop to Laboratory, June 1873–March 1876.* Ed. Reese V. Jenkins. Baltimore: Johns Hopkins University Press.

Edlin, J.V. (1942). Electrically Induced Convulsions for the Treatment of Functional Psychoses. *Illinois Medical Journal* 81:216–222.

Elfeld, P.F. (1941). Electric Shock Therapy. *Delaware State Medical Journal* 13 (June):95–98.

Endler, N. (1982). *Holiday of Darkness: A Psychologist's Personal Journey Out of His Own Depression.* New York: John Wiley & Sons.

———. (1988a). The Origins of Electroconvulsive Therapy. *Convulsive Therapy* 4:5–23.

———. (1988b). *Electroconvulsive Therapy: The Myths and Realities.* Toronto: Hans Huber.

Erb, W. (1883). *Handbook of Electro-Therapeutics.* Translated by L. Putzel. New York: William Wood and Co.

Essid, J. (1993). No God But Electricity: American Literature and Technological Enthusiasm in the Electrical Age. Unpublished diss., Indiana University.

Everts (1880). Dr. G.M. Beard on Insanity. *American Journal of Insanity* 37:229–236.

Ewalt, J.R., & Ewalt, P.L. (1969). History of the Community Psychiatry Movement. *American Journal of Psychiatry* 126:43–52.

Farber, S. (1991). Romancing Electroshock. *Z Magazine,* June, 92–99.

———. (1995). Electroconvulsive Therapy Is Harmful. In *Mental Illness: Opposing Viewpoints,* ed. D. Bender and B. Leone. San Diego: Greenhaven Press.

Feldman, F., Susselman, S., Lipetz, B., & Barrera, S.E. (1946). Electric Shock Therapy of Elderly Patients. *Archives of Neurology and Psychiatry* 56:158–170.

Felix, R. (1949). Introduction. In *The Mentally Ill in America,* ed. A. Deutsch. New York: Columbia University Press.

Ferguson, J. (1775). *An Introduction to Electricity, in Six Sections*. London: W. Strahan and T. Cadell.

Fetterman, J.L. (1942). Electro-Shock Therapy. *Ohio State Medical Journal* 38:675–676.

Fink, M. (1985). Convulsive Therapy. Letters to the Editor. *Convulsive Therapy* 1:1–3.

———. (1988). Use of ECT in the United States. *American Journal of Psychiatry* 145:133–134.

———. (1989). News and Notes. *Convulsive Therapy* 5:199.

———. (1991). Impact of the Antipsychiatry Movement on the Revival of Electroconvulsive Therapy in the United States. *Psychiatric Clinics of North America* 14:793–801.

———. (1994a). Frank Gagliardi. *Convulsive Therapy* 10:67.

———. (1994b). New Estimates of ECT Use in the United States. *Convulsive Therapy* 10:242.

———. (1997). What Is the Role of ECT in Mania? *Harvard Mental Health Letter* (June):8.

———. (1999). *Electroshock: Restoring the Mind*. New York: Oxford University Press.

———. (2000). Electroshock Revisited. *American Scientist* 88, March, 162–167.

Fink, M., & Bailine, S.H. (1998). Electroconvulsive Therapy and Managed Care. *Journal of Managed Care* 4:107–112.

Fleischbacker, H.H. (1945). Some Neurological and Neurovegetative Phenomena Occurring During and After Electroshock. *Journal of Nervous and Mental Disease* 102:185–189.

Flint, A., Jr. (1874). *The Physiology of Man*. Vol. 5, *Special Senses: Generation*. New York: D. Appleton and Co.

Foderaro, L.W. (1993). With Reforms in Treatment, Shock Therapy Loses Shock. *New York Times*, 19 July, A1, A11.

Foucault, M. (1973). *Madness and Civilization: A History of Insanity in the Age of Reason*. Translated by R. Howard. New York: Vintage.

Frank, L.R. (1978). *The History of Shock Treatment*. San Francisco: Leonard Roy Frank.

———. (1990). Electroshock: Death, Brain Damage, Memory Loss, and Brainwashing. *Journal of Mind and Behavior* 11:489–512.

Frankel, F. (1982). Medicolegal and Ethical Aspects of Treatment. In *Electroconvulsive Therapy: Biological Foundations and Clinical Applications*, ed. R. Abrams and B. Essman. New York: Spectrum Publications.

———. (1975). Reasoned Discourse or a Holy War?: Postscript to a Report on ECT. *American Journal of Psychiatry* 132:77–79.

———. (1977). Current Perspectives on ECT: A Discussion. *American Journal of Psychiatry* 134:1014–1019.

Franklin, B. (1961). *The Papers of Benjamin Franklin*, ed. Leonard Labaree. Vol. 4. New Haven: Yale University Press.

———. (1962). *The Papers of Benjamin Franklin*, ed. Leonard Labaree. Vol. 5. New Haven: Yale University Press.

Freedman, A.M., Kaplan, H.I., & Sadock, B.J. (1975). *Comprehensive Textbook of Psychiatry*. Vol. 1. 2nd ed. William S. Wilkins Co.

Freeman, L. (1953). *Hope for the Troubled*. New York: Crown.

———. (1956). Out of Darkness. *The Nation*, 3 March, 255.

Friedberg, J. (1975a). Electroconvulsive Therapy: Let's Stop Blasting the Brain. *Psychology Today* 9 (August):1–23, 98–99.

———. (1975b). Letters: John Freidberg Replies. *Psychology Today* 10 (December):8, 13, 106.

———. (1976). *Shock Treatment Is Not Good for Your Brain.* San Francisco: Glide Publications.

———. (1977). Shock Treatment: Brain Damage and Memory Loss: A Neurology Perspective. *American Journal of Psychiatry* 134:1010–1014.

Friedman, E. (1942). Unidirectional Electrostimulated Convulsive Therapy. *American Journal of Psychiatry* 99 (September):218–223.

Friedman, L.J. (1990). *The Menningers: The Family and the Clinic.* Lawrence: University of Kansas Press.

Gale, T. (1802). *Electricity: Or Ethereal Fire Considered.* Troy: Moffit and Lyon.

Galt, J. (1870). Hospital and Cottage Systems for the Care of the Insane. *American Journal of Insanity* 27:80–101.

Galvano-Faradic Co. (1891). *Illustrated Catalog.* Rahway, NJ: Mershan Press.

Gaspar, D., & Samarasinghe, L.A. (1982). ECT in Psychogeriatric Practice—A Study of Risk Factors, Indications, and Outcomes. *Comprehensive Psychiatry* 23:170–175.

Gelman, D., Hager, M., Doherty, S., Gosenell, M., Raine, G., & Shapiro, D. (1987). Depression. *Newsweek,* 4 May, 48–57.

Gilbert, W. (1600). *De Magnete.* London: P. Short.

Goelet, A. (1893). Influences Governing the Progress of Electro-Therapeutics. *Transactions of the American Electrotherapeutic Association* 3:1–3.

Goffman, E. (1961). *Asylums: Essays on the Social Situation of Mental Patients and Other Inmates.* Garden City, NY: Doubleday.

Goldman, D. (1949). Brief Stimulus Electric Shock Therapy. *Journal of Nervous and Mental Diseases* 110:36–45.

Goldman, D., & Baber, E.A. (1942). Electric Convulsive Therapy in Psychoses. *American Journal of Medical Science* 203:354–359.

Gonda, V.E. (1941). Treatment of Mental Disorders with Electrically Induced Convulsions. *Diseases of the Nervous System* 2:84–92.

Gordon, H.L. (1948). Fifty Shock Therapy Theories. *Military Surgeon* 103:397–401.

Gralnick, A. (1945). A Fatality Incident to Electroshock Treatment. *Journal of Nervous and Mental Diseases* 102:483–495.

Granger, F. (1920). Electrotherapy and Physiology in the Medical School. *American Journal of Electrotherapeutics and Radiology* 38:448.

Gray, J.P. (1871). The Dependence of Insanity on Physical Disease. *American Journal of Insanity* 27:377–408.

Green, H. (1986). *Fit for America: Health, Fitness, Sport, and American Society.* New York: Pantheon Books.

Greenblatt, M. (1955). Toward a Therapeutic Community. In *From Custodial to Therapeutic Patient Care in Mental Hospitals: Explorations in Social Treatment,* ed. M. Greenblatt, R. York, and F.L. Brown. New York: Russell Sage Foundation.

———. (1984a). Editorial Introduction: Electroconvulsive Therapy: A Problem in Social Psychiatry. *American Journal of Social Psychiatry* 4 (fall):3–5.

———. (1984b). ECT: Please No More Regulation. *American Journal of Psychiatry* 141:1409–1410.

Greenway, J.L. (1989). Nervous Disease and Electric Medicine. In *Pseudo-Sciences and Society in the Nineteenth Century,* ed. Arthur Wrobel. Kentucky: University Press of Kentucky.

Grob, G. (1962). Samuel Woodward and the Practice of Psychiatry in Early Nine-teenth-Century America. *Bulletin of the History of Medicine* 36:420–443.

———. (1977). Rediscovering Asylums: The Unhistorical History of the Mental Hospital. *Hastings Center Report* 7:33–41.

———. (1983). *Mental Illness in America, 1875–1940*. Princeton, NJ: Princeton University Press.

———. (1991). *From Asylum to Community: Mental Health Policy in Modern America*. Princeton, NJ: Princeton University Press.

———. (1994). *The Mad Among Us: A History of the Care of America's Mentally Ill*. New York: Free Press.

Gronner R. (1945). Comments Upon the Dynamics and Results of Electric Shock Treatment. *Elgin State Paper* 5:63–70.

Grosser, G.H. et al. (1975). The Regulation of Electroconvulsive Treatment in Massachusetts: A Follow Up Report. *Massachusetts Journal of Mental Health* 5:12–25.

Gumplowicz, M., & Klotzberg, E. (1874). Report of the Results of Electrical Treatment As Administered in the Department for Nervous Diseases and Electro-Therapeutics of the General Hospital in Vienna. *The Chicago Journal* 1:317–363.

Hale, N. (1995). *The Rise and Crisis of Psychoanalysis in the United States: Freud and the Americans, 1917–1985*. New York: Oxford University Press.

Haller, J.S. (1971). Neurasthenia, the Medical Profession, and the New Woman of the Late Nineteenth Century. *New York State Journal of Medicine* 71:469–474.

———. (1985). Medical Cataphoresis: Electrical Experimentation and Nineteenth Century Therapeutics. *New York State Journal of Medicine* 85:257–261.

Hammond, W.A. (1871). *A Treatise on the Diseases of the Nervous System*. New York: D. Appleton.

Hankins, T. (1985). *Science and the Enlightenment*. New York: Cambridge University Press.

Hanson, A.E., & King, H. (1995). Greek and Roman Gynecology. *Society for Ancient Medicine* 23 (December):94–99.

Harman, P.M. (1982). *Energy, Force, and Matter: The Conceptual Development of Nineteenth Century Physics*. Cambridge: Cambridge University Press.

Harms, E. (1955). The Origins and Early History of Electrotherapy and Electro-shock. *American Journal of Psychiatry* 111:933–934.

Hauser, A., & Barbato, L. (1941). Electric Shock Therapy. *Texas State Journal of Medicine* 37 (July):228–233.

Hay, D., Hay, L., & Spiro, H. (1989). The Enigma of the Stigma of ECT: 50 Years of Myth and Misrepresentation. *Wisconsin Medical Journal* 88:4–10.

Hay, D.P. (1992). The Stigma of Electroconvulsive Therapy: A Workshop. In *Stigma and Mental Illness*, ed. P.J. Fink and A. Tasman. Washington, D.C.: American Psychiatric Press.

Haygarth, J. (1800). Of the Imagination, As a Cause and As a Cure of Disorders of the Body; Exemplified by Fictitious Tractors and Epidemical Convulsions. Read to the Literary and Philosophical Society of Bath. Printed by R. Curtwell, Bath.

Health Reporter. (1995). Crosscurrents. *Mirabella*, 70, 169–171.

Hedley, W.S. (1900). *Therapeutic Electricity and Practical Muscle Testing*. Philadelphia: P. Blakiston's Son and Co.

Heilbron, J.L. (1979). *Electricity in the 17th and 18th Centuries: A Study of Early Modern Physics*. Berkeley: University of California Press.

Herbert, W. (1982). Berkeley Voters Ban ECT, Shock Psychiatric Profession. *Science News* 122 (13 November):309.

Herbert, W. (1983). ECT Ban Banned. *Science News* 123 (29 January):71.

Hippocrates, I. (1923). Translated and edited by W.H.S. Jones. Cambridge, MA: Harvard University Press.

Hippocrates, II. (1931). Translated and edited by W.H.S. Jones. Cambridge, MA: Harvard University Press.

Holden, C. (1985). A Guarded Endorsement for Shock Therapy. *Science* 228:55.

Horn D. (1994). *Social Bodies: Reproductive Technology and Italian Modernity*. Princeton, NJ: Princeton University Press.

Hughes, T.P. (1989). *American Genesis: A Century of Invention and Technological Enthusiasm, 1870–1970*. New York: Penguin Books.

Hunter, R., & Macalpine, I. (1963). *Three Hundred Years of Psychiatry, 1535–1860*. London: Oxford University Press.

Hutchins, R. (1939). Presidential Address. *American Journal of Psychiatry* 96:1–14.

Hutchinson, W.F. (1875). Hysteria and Spinal Irritation Treated by Central Galvanization. *Archives of Electrology and Neurology* 1:62.

Hyde, A. (1975). ECT Malpractice Insurance. *Convulsive Therapy Bulletin with Tardive Dyskinesia Notes*, 2, 46.

Impastato, B.S., & Gabriel, A. (1957). The Molac II: An Alternating Current Electroshock Therapy Machine Incorporating a New Principle. *Journal of Nervous and Mental Diseases* 125:380–384.

Impastato, D. (1960). The Story of the First Electroshock Treatment. *American Journal of Psychiatry* 116:1113–1114.

International Correspondence School. (1903). *A System of Electrotherapeutics*. Scranton, PA: ICS.

Isaac, R.J., & Armat, V. (1990). *Madness in the Streets: How Psychiatry and the Law Abandoned the Mentally Ill*. New York: Free Press.

———. (1995). Electroconvulsive Therapy Is Safe. In *Mental Illness: Opposing Viewpoints*, ed. D. Bender and B. Leone. San Diego: Greenhaven Press.

Ives, J. (1879). *Electricity As a Medicine and its Mode of Application*. New York: John T. Ives, Jr.

Jackson, W.L. (1895). The Development of Electrotherapeutics and Its Relation to the Practice of Medicine. *Transactions of the National Society of Electrotherapeutists* 3:1–6.

Jacobi, M.P. (1888). *Essays on Hysteria, Brain Tumors, and Some Other Cases of Nervous Diseases*. New York: G.P. Putnam's Sons.

Janis, I. (1950a). Psychological Effects of Electrical Convulsive Treatments. *Journal of Nervous and Mental Diseases* 111:359–382.

———. (1950b). Psychological Effects of Electric Convulsive Treatments, II (Changes in Word Association Reactions). *Journal of Nervous and Mental Diseases* 111:383–397.

Jardine, L. (1999). *Ingenious Pursuits: Building the Scientific Revolution*. New York: Nan A. Talese.

Jefferson, J.W. (1983). Treating Affective Disorders in the Presence of Cardiovascular Disease. *Psychiatric Clinics of North America* 6:141–155.

Jewell, J.S., & Bannister, H.M. (1874a). Therapeutics of the Nervous System and Mind. *The Chicago Journal of Nervous and Mental Diseases* 1:100–107.

———. (1874b). Review of Recent Works in Medical Electricity. *The Chicago Journal of Nervous and Mental Diseases* 1:208–215.

Joerges, B. (1990). Images of Technology in Sociology: Computer As Butterfly and Bat. *Technology and Culture* 31:203–227.

Jones, H.L. (1901). The Use of General Electrification As Means of Treatment in Certain Forms of Disease. *Journal of Mental Science* 47:245–250.

Jordanova, L. (1989). *Sexual Visions: Images of Gender in Science and Medicine Between the Eighteenth and Twentieth Centuries*. Madison: University of Wisconsin Press.

Kalayam, B., & Steinhart, M.J. (1981). A Survey of Attitudes on the Use of Electro-convulsive Therapy. *Hospital and Community Psychiatry* 32:185–188.

Kalinowsky, L. (1948). Failures with Electric Shock Therapy. In *Failures in Psychiatric Treatment*, ed. P. Hoch. New York: Grune and Stratton.

———. (1959). Electroshock. In *American Handbook of Psychiatry*, ed. S. Arieti. Vol. 2. New York: Basic Books.

———. (1982). The History of Electroconvulsive Therapy. In *Electroconvulsive Therapy: Biological Foundations and Clinical Applications*, ed. R. Abrams and W. Essman. New York: Spectrum Publications.

Kalinowsky, L., & Hoch, P. (1946). *Shock Treatments and Other Somatic Procedures in Psychiatry*. New York: Grune and Stratton.

Karasu, T. (1984). *Psychiatric Therapies*. Washington, D.C.: American Psychiatric Association.

Katz, J. (1975). *Psychoanalysis, Psychiatry, and the Law*. New York: Free Press.

———. (1976). *Gay American History: Lesbians and Gay Men in the USA*. New York: Thomas Y. Crowell.

Kavy, W.H. (1965). *We Can't All Be Sane*. Los Angeles: Collector's Publishing.

Keisler, C., & Sibulkin, A.E. (1987). *Mental Hospitalization: Myths and Facts About a National Crisis*. Beverly Hills, CA: Sage.

Kellaway, P. (1946). The Part Played by Electric Fish in the Early History of Bio-electricity and Electrotherapy. *Bulletin of the History of Medicine* 20:112–137.

Kellner, C. (1991). Electroconvulsive Therapy. *The Psychiatric Clinics of North America* 14:793–1016.

Kennedy, J.F. (1964). Message from the President of the United States Relative to Mental Illness and Mental Retardation. *American Journal of Psychiatry* 120:729–737.

Kesey, K. (1962). *One Flew Over the Cuckoo's Nest*. New York: Viking Press.

King, H. (1993). Once Upon a Text: Hysteria from Hippocrates. In *Hysteria Beyond Freud*, ed. S.L. Gilman, H. King, R. Porter, G.S. Rousseau, and E. Showalter. Berkeley: University of California Press.

King, W.H. (1892). Quackery and Electrotherapy. *Journal of Electrotherapeutics* 10:43.

———. (1901). *Electricity in Medicine and Surgery, Including the X-Ray*. New York: Boericke and Runyon.

Klein, D., & Wender, P. (1993). *Understanding Depression: A Complete Guide to Its Diagnosis and Treatment*. New York: Oxford University Press.

Kneeland, T.W. (1996). *The Use of Electricity to Treat Mental Illness in the United States, 1870 to the Present*. Unpublished diss. University of Oklahoma.

Kolb, L., & Rolzin, L. (1993). *The First Psychiatric Institute*. Washington, D.C.: American Psychiatric Association.

Kolb, L., & Vogel, V. (1942). The Use of Shock Therapy in 305 Mental Hospitals. *American Journal of Psychiatry* 99:90–100.

Kovacs, R. (1925). Let There Be a Section of Physical Therapy in the American Medical Association. *Physical Therapeutics* 43:313–316.

———. (1932). *Electrotherapy and the Elements of Light Therapy*. Philadelphia: Lea and Febiger.

Kramer, M.B. (1977). *Psychiatric Services and the Changing Institutional Scene*, DHEW Publication (ADM) 77–433. Washington, D.C.: Government Printing Office.

———. (1985). The Use of ECT in California, 1977–1983. *American Journal of Psychiatry* 142:1190–1192.

———. (1999). ECT Use in the Public Sector: California. *Psychiatric Quarterly* 61:97–103.

Krusen, F.H. (1942). *Physical Medicine: The Employment of Physical Agents for Diagnosis and Therapy*. Philadelphia: W.B. Saunders.

Kuhfeld, A. (1992). The Life and Times of Victor Frankenstein. *Engineering in Medicine and Biology* (June):68–69.

Laing, R.D. (1969). *Self and Others*. 2nd ed. New York: Penguin.

Laqueur, T. (1990). *Making Sex: Body and Gender from the Greeks to Freud*. Cambridge, MA: Harvard University Press.

Lasch, C. (1979). *The Culture of Narcissism: American Life in an Age of Diminishing Expectations*. New York: W.W. Norton.

Lebensohn, Z. (1984). Electroconvulsive Therapy: Psychiatry's Villain or Hero? *The American Journal of Social Psychiatry* 4 (fall):39–43.

Lee, B. (1881). Swedish Movements and Massage. In *A System of Practical Therapeutics*, ed. H.A. Hare. Vol. 1. Philadelphia: Lea Bros.

Lehmann, H.L. (1982). Affective Disorders in the Aged. *Psychiatric Clinics of North America* 5:27–48.

Lewis, N.D.C., & Engle, B., eds. (1954). *Wartime Psychiatry: A Compendium of the International Literature*. New York: Oxford University Press.

Libbrecht, K., & Quackenbush, J. (1995). On the Early History of Male Hysteria and Psychic Trauma. *Journal of the History of the Behavioral Sciences* 31:370–384.

Licht, S. (1967). *Therapeutic Electricity and Ultraviolet Radiation*. Baltimore: Waverly Press.

Lidz, C.W., Meisel, A., Zerubavel, E., Carter, M., Sestak, R.M., & Roth, L. (1981). *Informed Consent: A Study of Decision-Making in Psychiatry*. New York: Guilford Press.

Linn, L. (1955). *A Handbook of Hospital Psychiatry: A Practical Guide to Therapy*. New York: International Universities Press.

Livingston, A.T. (1898). Electrotherapeutics in Insanity. *Transactions of the Annual Meeting of the American Electrotherapeutic Association* 8:342–351.

Livingston, J.D. (2000). An Electromagnetic Personality. *Nature* 407:453.

Lloyd, G.E.R. (1973). *Greek Science After Aristotle*. New York: W.W. Norton.

Logan, K. (1995). *The Use of ECT with Children and Adolescents*. Mayo Clinic publication.

Longo, L.D. (1979). The Rise and Fall of Battey's Operation: A Fashion in Surgery. *Bulletin of the History of Medicine* 53:244–267.

———. (1986). Electrotherapy in Gynecology: The American Experience. *Bulletin of the History of Medicine* 60:343–366.

Lovett, R. (1756). *The Subtil Medium Proved*. London: Hinton, Sandby and Lovett.

Lowenbach, H. (1943). Electric Shock Treatment of Mental Disorders. *North Carolina Medical Journal* 4:123–128.

Lowndes, F. (1787). *Observations on Medical Electricity*. London: D. Stuart.

Lunbeck, E. (1994). *The Psychiatric Persuasion: Knowledge, Gender and Power in Modern America*. Princeton, NJ: Princeton University Press.

Mackay, C. (1841). *Memoirs of Extraordinary Popular Delusions*. Vol. 1. London: Richard Bentley.

Macklis, R.M. (1993). Magnetic Healing, Quackery, and the Debate About Health Effects of Electron Fields. *Annals of Internal Medicine* 118 (1 March):376–383.

Maines, R. (1989). Socially Camouflaged Technology. *IEEE Technology and Society Magazine* 8 (June):3–23.

———. (1999). *The Technology of Orgasm*. Baltimore: Johns Hopkins University Press.

Maisel, A. (1946). Bedlam 1946. *Life* (May):102–118.

Manning, M. (1994). *Undercurrents: A Therapist's Reckoning with Her Own Depression*. New York: Harper.

———. (1995). Crosscurrents. *Mirabella* (March):169–171.

Martin, W. (1920). Oral Infections and Mental Diseases. *American Journal of Electrotherapeutics and Radiology* 38 (April):151.

Massey, G.B. (1889). *Report of Recent Electrotherapeutic Work of Dr. G. Betton Massey's Private Hospital*. Philadelphia: G. Betton Massey.

May, E.T. (1988). *Homeward Bound*. New York: Basic Books.

Mayer, W. (1991). *1990 Electroconvulsive Therapy (ECT) Report*. California: Department of Mental Health.

McGinnes, E. (1894). The Use of Electricity in Obstetrics; Galactorrhoea; Sore Nippleism. In *An International System of Electro-Therapeutics*, ed. H.R. Bigelow. Philadelphia: F.A. Davis Co.

McGovern, C. (1985). *Masters of Madness: The Social Origins of the American Psychiatric Profession*. Hanover, NH: University Press of New England.

McIntosh Battery. (1914). *Electrotherapeutics Catalogue: Everything Electrotherapeutical*. 32nd ed. Chicago: McIntosh Battery.

Meduna, L.J. (1954). The Convulsive Treatment: A Reappraisal. *Journal of Clinical and Experimental Psychopathology and Quarterly Review of Psychiatry and Neurology* 15:215–254.

Meigs, C.D. (1851). *Woman: Her Diseases and Remedies*. 2nd rev. ed. Philadelphia: Lea and Blanchard.

Menninger, W.C. (1947). Psychiatric Experience in the War, 1941–1946. *American Journal of Psychiatry* 103:577–586.

———. (1948). *Psychiatry in a Troubled World: Yesterday's War and Today's Challenge*. New York: Macmillan.

Meyers, B.S., & Mei-Tal, V. (1985). Empirical Study of an Inpatient Psychogeriatric Unit: Biological Treatment in Patients with Depressive Illness. *International Journal of Psychiatry in Medicine* 15:111–174.

Mielke, D.H., Winstead, D.K., Goethe, J.W., & Schwartz, B.D. (1984). Multiple-Monitored Electroconvulsive Therapy: Safety and Efficacy in Elderly Depressed Patients. *Journal of the American Geriatrics Society*, 32(3):180–182.

Milledgeville State Hospital. (1951). *One Hundred Ninth Annual Report*. Milledgeville, GA.

Millet, A.P., & Mosse, E.P. (1944). Psychosomatic Medicine. Reprinted in *Abstracts and Translations from the Science Library*. Series XII. Hartford, CT: Institute of Living.

Milling, C. (1943). Observations in Shock Therapy. *The Journal of the South Carolina Medical Association* 39:182–187.

Mitchell, S.W. (1885). *Fat and Blood: An Essay on the Treatment of Certain Forms of Neurasthenia and Hysteria*. 4th ed. Philadelphia: J.B. Lippincott.

———. (1894). Address to the Fiftieth Annual Meeting. *Journal of Nervous and Mental Diseases* 21:413–437.

Molle, A.S. (1975). ECT in the Home. *Convulsive Therapy Bulletin with Tardive Dyskinesia Notes* 1:20–21.

Monell, S.E. (1871). Therapeutic Electricity. *Eclectic Medical Journal* 31:110–112.

Monell, S.H. (1910). *High Frequency Electric Currents in Medicine and Dentistry*. New York: W. Jenkins Co.

Morey, L.G. (1882). *Catalogue and Price List of Electrical Apparatus and Supplies*. Philadelphia: author.

Moriarity, J.D. (1953). Technique of Electro-Stimulative Therapy in Office Practice. *Confinia Neurologia* 13:333–339.

Morrisey, J.P., Burton, N.M., & Steadman, H.J. (1979). Developing an Empirical Base for Psycho-Legal Policy Analyses of ECT: A New York State Survey. *International Journal of Law and Psychiatry* 2:99–111.

Morrissey, J.E., Steadman, H.J., & Burton, N. (1981). A Profile of ECT Recipients in New York State During 1972 and 1977. *American Journal of Psychiatry* 138:618–622.

Morse, W.N. (1934). Lectures on Electricity in Colonial Times. *The New England Quarterly* 7:264–374.

Morrill, S.E. (1871). Therapeutic Electricity. *Eclectic Medical Journal* 31:110–112.

Morton, W.J. (1892). Electricity and Medicinal Art and Science. *Transactions of the American Electrotherapeutical Association* 2:2–4.

Morus, I.R. (1992). Marketing the Machine: The Construction of Electrotherapeutics As Viable Medicine in Early Victorian England. *Medical History* 36:34–52.

———. (1993). Currents from the Underworld: Electricity and the Technology of Display in Early Victorian England. *Isis* 84:50–69.

Murray, J.A.H., ed. (1885). *The New English Dictionary*. Vol. 1. Oxford: Clarendon Press.

Myerson, A. (1942). Further Experience with Electric Shock Therapy in Mental Disease. *New England Journal of Medicine* 227:403–407.

Myerson, A., Feldman L., & Green, I. (1941). Experience with Electric Shock Therapy in Mental Disease. *New England Journal of Medicine* 224:1081–1085.

Napheys, G.H. (1875). *The Physical Life of Woman: Advice to the Maiden, Wife, and Mother*. 5th ed. Philadelphia: Fergus, Watts & Co.

Neaman, J. (1976). *Suggestion of the Devil*. New York: Hippocrene Books.

Neff, I. (1896). Uses of Electricity in the Treatment of Insanity. *American Journal of Insanity* 53:322–324.

Neiswanger, C.S. (1900). The Value of Primary Education in Electro-Therapeutics. *The Electro-Therapeutist* 3:31–32.

———. (1906). *Electrotherapeutic Practice: A Ready Reference Guide for Physicians in the Use of Electricity*. 15th ed. Chicago: Ritchie and Co.

Nelson, P. (1973). History of the Once Close Relationship Between Electrotherapeutics and Radiology. *Archives of Physical Medicine and Rehabilitation* 54 (December): 608–640.

Neoforma. (1999). ECT Units. Available online at http://www.neoforma.net.

Network Against Psychiatric Assault. (1975). *Shock Packet.* n.p.

Newman, R. (1896). The Want of College Instruction in Electro-Therapeutics. *Transaction of the American Electrotherapeutic Association* 6:25–32.

Neymann, C., Urse, V.G., Madden, J., & Countryman, M.A. (1943). Electric Shock Therapy in the Treatment of Schizophrenia, Manic Depressive Psychoses and Chronic Alcoholism. *The Journal of Nervous and Mental Diseases* 98:618–637.

Nordenberg, L. (1998). Dealing with the Depths of Depression. *FDA Consumer* 32 (19 August):n.p.

North, E. (1991). An Old Therapy Brings New Hope. *Menninger Perspective* 22:5–7.

Nye, D. (1991). *Electrifying America: Social Meanings of a New Technology, 1880–1940.* Cambridge, MA: MIT Press.

O'Brien, D.R. (1989). The Effective Agent in Electroconvulsive Therapy: Convulsion or Coma? *Medical Hypotheses* 28:277–280.

Otis, W.J. (1941–1942). Electro-Shock Therapy. *New Orleans Medical and Surgical Journal* 94:239–242.

Overmeier, J., & Senior, J. (1992). *Books and Manuscripts of the Bakken.* Metuchen, NJ: Scarecrow Press.

Ozarin, L.D. (1993). The First Use of ECT in the United States. *Psychiatric News* 16 (August):15.

Pace, E. (1992). Lothar Kalinowsky. *New York Times* 141 (30 June):D23.

Pallanti, S. (1999). Images in Psychiatry: Ugo Cerletti, 1877–1963. *American Journal of Psychiatry* 156:630.

Palmer, R., ed. (1981). *Electroconvulsive Therapy: An Appraisal.* New York: Oxford University Press.

Paramore, R.H. (1921). The Neurasthenic Element in Mid-Wifery and Gynecology. *British Medical Journal* 11:768–769.

Paul, F. (1942). Observations Concerning Electroshock Therapy. *Delaware State Medical Journal* 12:86–88.

Pearlman, C. (1991). Electroconvulsive Therapy: Current Concepts. *General Hospital Psychiatry* 13:128–137.

Peck, R. (1974). *The Miracle of Shock Treatment.* New York: Jericho Press.

Perkins, B.D. (1799). *Experiments with the Metallic Tractors.* London: Luke Hanford.

Peterson, M.C., & Turner, T.R. (1943). Electric Convulsive Therapy of Mental Disease. *Medical Clinics of North America* 27:1019–1023.

Pettinanti, H.M., Bonner, K.M. (1984). Cognitive Functioning in Depressed Geriatric Patients with a History of ECT. *American Journal of Psychiatry* 141:49–52.

Phelps, O.S. (1894). Some Landmarks in Electro-Therapeutics. *Transactions of the American Electrotherapeutic Association* 2:3.

Philadelphia Psychiatric Society (1943). Symposium: Complications of and Contradictions to Electrical Shock Therapy. *Archives of Neurology and Psychiatry* 49:786–791.

Plath, S. (1968). Johnny Panic and the Bible of Dreams. *Atlantic Monthly*, September, 54–60.

———. (1971). *The Bell Jar.* New York: Harper and Row.

Poinar, G.O., Jr. (1992). *Life in Amber*. Stanford, CA: Stanford University Press.

Poirer, S. (1983). The Weir Mitchell Rest Cure: Doctor and Patient. *Women's Studies* 10:15–40.

Polatin, P. (1945). Shock Therapy in Schizophrenia. *The Family: Journal of Social Case Work* 26:283–289.

———. (1946). Shock Therapy in Psychiatry. *The Family: Journal of Social Case Work* 27:174–177.

Polatin, P., & Philtine, E. (1949). *How Psychiatry Helps*. New York: Harper and Row.

Popenoe, P. (1952). *Marriage Is What You Make It*. New York: Macmillan.

Porter, R. (1989). *Health for Sale: Quackery in England, 1660–1850*. Manchester: Manchester University Press.

———. (1991). *The Faber Book of Madness*. London: Faber.

Porter, R., & Hall, L. (1996). *The Facts of Life: The Creation of Sexual Knowledge in Britain, 1650–1950*. New Haven, CT: Yale University Press.

Pressman, J. (1998). *Last Resort: Psychosurgery and the Limits of Medicine*. New York: Cambridge University Press.

Pring, J.N. (1929). Electrotherapy. *The Encyclopædia Britannica*. Vol. 8. 14th ed. London: Britannica.

Pulver, S.E. (1961). The First Electroconvulsive Treatment Given in the United States. *American Journal of Psychiatry* 117:845–846.

Rael, I., & Armat, V. (1990). *Madness in the Streets: How Psychiatry and the Law Abandoned the Ill*. New York: Free Press.

Ray, M.B. (1946). *Doctors of the Mind: What Psychiatry Can Do*. Rev. ed. Boston: Little Brown, & Co.

Read, C. (1945). *Elgin Papers*. Vol. 5. Elgin, IL: Elgin State Hospital.

Reismann, J.M. (1976). *A History of Clinical Psychology*. New York: Irvington.

Reynolds, E. (1910). Gynecological Operations on Neurasthenics: Advantages, Disadvantages, Selected Cases. *Boston Medical and Surgical Journal* CCXIII:113–117.

Rickles, N.K., & Olson, C. (1948). Causes of Failure in Treatment with Electric Shock. *Archives of Neurology and Psychiatry* 59:337–346.

Riddle, J.M. (1992a). Amber in Ancient Pharmacy. *Quid Pro Quo: Studies in the History of Drugs*. Brookfield, VT: Ashfield Publishing Co.

———. (1992b). Pomum Ambrae: Amber and Ambergris in Plague Remedies. *Quid Pro Quo: Studies in the History of Drugs*. Brookfield, VT: Ashgate Publishing Co.

Ripa, Y. (1990). *Women and Madness: The Incarceration of Women in Nineteenth Century France*. Minneapolis: University of Minnesota Press.

Roan, S. (1992). A New Image for Shock Therapy. *Los Angeles Times*, 15 September, E1–4.

Roback, A.A., Keirnan, T., eds. (1969). *Pictorial History of Psychology and Psychiatry*. New York: Philosophical Library.

Robinson, W.F. (1892). *Electrotherapeutics of Neurasthenia*. Detroit: G & S Davis.

Robitscher, J. (1980). *The Powers of Psychiatry*. Boston: Houghton Mifflin.

Roccatagliata, G. (1986). *A History of Ancient Psychiatry*. Westport, CT: Greenwood Press.

Rockwell, A.D. (1891). Electro-Therapeutics. In *A System of Practical Therapeutics*, ed. H.A. Hare. Vol. 1. Philadelphia: Lea Brothers.

———. (1920). *Rambling Recollections: An Autobiography*. New York: Paul Hoeber.

Rosenberg, C. (1962). The Place of George M. Beard in Nineteenth-Century Psychiatry. *Bulletin of the History of Medicine* 36:245–259.

Roth, N. (1977). The Nineteenth-Century Revival of Electrotherapy. *Medical Instrumentation* 11:236–237.

———. (1981). Electrotherapy, 19th Century Neurasthenia, and the Case of Alice James. *Medical Instrumentation* 15:111.

Rothman, D. (1971). *The Discovery of the Asylum: Social Order and Disorder in the New Republic.* Boston: Little, Brown and Co.

Rowbottom, M., & Susskind, C. (1984). *Electricity and Medicine: A History of Their Interaction.* San Francisco: San Francisco Press.

Rudloe, A., & Rudloe, J. (1993). Electric Warfare: The Fish That Kill with Thunderbolts. *The Smithsonian* 24:94–105.

Russell, R.W., Pierce, J.F., Rohrer, W.M., & Townsend, J.C. (1948). A New Apparatus for the Controlled Administration of Electroconvulsive Shock. *The Journal of Psychology* 26:71–82.

Russell, W.L. (1945). *The New York Hospital: A History of the Psychiatric Service, 1771–1936.* New York: Columbia University Press.

Rydell, R. (1984). *All the World's a Fair: Visions of Empire at American International Expositions, 1876–1916.* Chicago: University of Chicago Press.

Sackeim, H. (1985). The Case for ECT. *Psychology Today* 19:36–40.

———. (1991). Are ECT Devices Underpowered? *Convulsive Therapy* 7:233–236.

Sakel, M. (1938). *The Pharmacological Shock Treatment of Schizophrenia.* New York: Nervous and Mental Disease Pub. Co., 1–13.

———. (1954). The Classical Sakel Shock Treatment. *Journal of Clinical and Experimental Psychopathology and Quarterly Review of Psychiatry and Neurology* 15:255–316.

Salzman, C. (1977). ECT and Ethical Psychiatry. *American Journal of Psychiatry* 134:1006–1009.

Sampson, H., Messinger, H.L., & Towne, R.D. (1964). *Schizophrenic Women: Studies in Marital Crisis.* New York: Paragon.

Schaffer, S. (1992). Self-Evidence. *Critical Inquiry* 18 (winter):327–336.

Schechter, D.C. (1983). *Exploring the Origins of Electrical Cardiac Stimulation.* Minneapolis, MN: Medtronic, Inc.

Schweig, G. (1876). Cerebral Exhaustion. *The Medical Record* 11:715–717.

———. (1877). *The Electric Bath.* New York: G.P. Putnam's Sons.

Scovern, A.W., & Kilman, P.R. (1980). Status of Electroconvulsive Therapy: A Review of Outcome Literature. *Psychological Bulletin* 87:260–303.

Scudder, J.M. (1898). *The American Eclectic: Materia Medica and Therapeutics.* 12th ed. Cincinnati: Scudder Bros.

Scull, A. (1987). Desperate Remedies: A Gothic Tale of Madness and Modern Medicine. *Psychological Medicine* 17:561–577.

Scull, A., & Favreau, D. (1986). A Chance to Cut Is a Chance to Cure: Sexual Surgery for Psychosis in Three Nineteenth Century Societies. In *Research in Law, Deviance and Social Control.* Vol. 8. London: JAI Press.

Scull, A., MacKenzie, C., & Hervey, N. (1996). *Masters of Bedlam: The Transformation of the Mad-Doctoring Trade.* Princeton, NJ: Princeton University Press.

Sears, Roebuck and Co. (1902). *Electrical Goods and Supplies.* Chicago: Sears.

Senior, J.E. (1983). The Magnet: Healing at a Distance. *Medical Instrumentation* 17 (6) (November–December):422.

Senter, N., Winsdale, W.J., Liston, E.H., & Mills, M.J. (1984). Electroconvulsive Therapy: The Evolution of Legal Regulation. *American Journal of Social Psychiatry* 4 (fall):11–15.

Shelley, M. (1817–1951). *Frankenstein or Modern Prometheus?* New York: Dell.

Shorter, E. (1985). *Bedside Manners: The Troubled History of Doctors and Patients.* New York: Simon & Schuster.

———. 1987). *The Health Century.* New York: Doubleday.

———. (1992). *From Paralysis to Fatigue: A History of Psychosomatic Illness in the Modern Era.* New York: Free Press.

———. (1994). *From the Mind into the Body: The Cultural Origins of Psychosomatic Symptoms.* New York: Free Press.

———. (1997). *A History of Psychiatry: From the Era of the Asylum to the Age of Prozac.* New York: John Wiley & Sons.

Showalter, E. (1985). *The Female Malady: Women, Madness, and English Culture, 1830–1980.* New York: Pantheon Books.

Shryock, H. (1947). Is Shock Treatment Successful? *Science Digest* 22 (October):60–65.

Sicherman, B. (1977). The Uses of Diagnosis: Doctors, Patients, and Neurasthenia. *Bulletin of the History of Medicine* 32:33–54.

Simon, B. (1978). *Mind and Madness in Ancient Greece: The Classical Roots of Modern Psychiatry.* Ithaca, NY: Cornell University Press.

Skultans, V. (1979). *English Madness: Ideas on Insanity, 1580–1890.* London: Routledge and Kegan Paul.

Slovenko, R. (1997). Highlights in the History of Law and Psychiatry with a Focus on the United States. *Journal of Psychiatry and Law* (winter):445–579.

Small, H. (1994). In the Guise of Science: Literature and the Rhetoric of 19th Century English Psychiatry. *History of the Human Sciences* 7:27–55.

Smee, A. (1849). *Elements of Electro-Biology.* London: Longman, Brown, Green and Longmans.

Smith, L.H., Hughes, J., & Hastings, D.W. (1941). First Impressions of Electroshock Treatment. *Pennsylvania Medical Journal* 44:452–455.

Snow, W.B. (1922). The Psychoneuroses Rarely of Purely Psychic Origin. *American Journal of Electrotherapeutics and Radiology* 40:60–61.

———. (1923). What Physical Therapeutics Constitutes. *American Journal of Electro-therapeutics and Radiology* 41:31–33.

———. (1925). Consideration of the Present Status of Physical Therapeutics. *American Journal of Electrotherapeutics and Radiology* 43:146–147.

———. (1928). Therapeutics of Neurology. *Physical Therapeutics* 46 (July):362–364.

Solomon, H.C., & Yakovlev, P.I., eds. (1944). *Manual of Military Neuropsychiatry.* Philadelphia: W.B. Saunders.

Solomon, J. (1996). Breaking the Silence. *Newsweek* 20 (May):20–22.

Somerville, W.G. (1916). The Psychology of Hysteria. *American Journal of Insanity* 73:639–653.

Spiegel, D. (1993). Introduction to the Progress on Psychiatry Series. *The Clinical Science of Electroconvulsive Therapy,* ed. Edward Coffey. Washington, D.C.: American Psychiatric Association.

Spurzeim, J.G. (1833). *Phrenology or the Doctrine of Mental Phenomena.* Boston: March, Capen & Lyon.

Squire, L.R., Slater, P.C., & Miller, P.L. (1981). Retrograde Amnesia and Bilateral Electroconvulsive Therapy, Long-Term Follow-Up. *Archives of General Psychiatry* 38:89–95.

Squire, S. (1987). Shock Therapy's Return to Respectability. *The New York Times Magazine* 22 November:78–79, 85, 88–89.

Stainbrook, E. (1948). The Use of Electricity in Psychiatric Treatment During the Nineteenth Century. *Bulletin of the History of Medicine* 22:156–177.

Staples, W.G. (1991). *Castles of our Conscience: Social Control and the American State, 1800–1985.* New Brunswick, NJ: Rutgers University Press.

Starr, P. (1982). *The Social Transformation of American Medicine.* New York: Basic Books.

Steele, A.J. (1871). *Theory and Practice of Electrical Therapeutics.* New York: American News Co.

Steinfeld, J.I. (1951). *Therapeutic Studies on Psychotics.* Des Plaines, IL: Forest Press.

Stephens, S., Greenberg, R., & Pettani, H.M. (1991). Choosing an Electroconvulsive Device. *Psychiatric Clinics of North America* 14 (December):989–1006.

Stephens, S., Pettinati, H.M., Greenberg, R.M., & Kelly, C.E. (1993). Continuation and Maintenance Therapy with Outpatient ECT. In *The Clinical Science of Electroconvulsive Therapy*, ed. E.C. Coffey. Progress in Psychiatry Series 38:143–164.

Stevens, R., & Stevens, R. (1974). *Welfare Medicine in America: A Case Study of Medicaid.* New York: The Free Press.

Stillings, D. (1983). Mediterranean Origins of Electrotherapy. *Journal of Bioelectricity* 2:181–186.

Stone, G. (1994). When Prozac Fails: Electroshock. *New York* 14 (November):55–59.

Strong, F.F. (1908). *High Frequency Currents.* New York: Rebman.

Stuart, H.R. (1889). *Our Family Physician.* New York: Smith and Hillman.

Sullivan-Fowler, M. (1995). Doubtful Theories, Drastic Therapies: Autointoxication and Faddism in the Late Nineteenth and Early Twentieth Centuries. *Journal of the History of Medicine and Allied Sciences* 50:364–390.

Sutton, G. (1981). Electric Medicine and Mesmerism. *Isis* 72:375–391.

Swayze, V. (1995). Frontal Leukotomy and Related Psychosurgical Procedures in the Era Before Antipsychotics (1935–1954): A Historical Overview. *American Journal of Psychiatry* 152:505–518.

Swazey, J.P. (1974). *Chlorpromazine in Psychiatry: A Study of Therapeutic Innovation.* Cambridge, MA: MIT Press.

Szasz, T. (1961). *The Myth of Mental Illness.* New York: Hoeber-Harper.

Tallack, D. (1991). *Twentieth-Century America: The Intellectual and Cultural Context.* New York: Longmans.

Taylor, E. (1983). The Electrified Hand: Therapeutic Implications. *Medical Instrumentation* 17 (July–August):281–282.

Taylor, R.W. (1905). *A Practical Treatise on Sexual Disorders of the Male and Female.* 3rd ed. New York: Lea Bros.

Temkin, O. (1971). *The Falling Sickness: A History of Epilepsy from the Greeks to the Beginnings of Modern Neurology.* 2nd ed. Baltimore: Johns Hopkins Press.

Thompson, J.W., & Blaine, J.D. (1987). Use of ECT in the U.S. in 1975 and 1980. *Journal of American Psychiatry* 144:557–562.

Thorndike, L. (1923). *A History of Magic and Experimental Science.* Vol. I. New York: Columbia University Press.

Tilney, F. (1924). What Neurology Needs from Physiotherapy. *American Journal of Electrotherapeutics and Radiology* 42 (January):57–64.

Tipton, A.W. (1882). *Electrical Medication*. Chicago: Chas. C. Johnson.

Tomes, N. (1984). *A Generous Confidence: Thomas Story Kirkbride and the Art of Asylum-Keeping, 1840–1883*. Cambridge: Cambridge University Press.

Tourney, G. (1971). History and Concepts of Schizophrenia. In *Lafayette Clinical Studies on Schizophrenia*, ed. G. Tourney and J.S. Gottlieb. Detroit: Wayne State University Press, 27–68.

Tousey, S. (1921). *Medical Electricity: Roentgen Rays and Radium*. 3rd ed. Philadelphia: W.B. Saunders.

Tripier, A. (1894). Engorgement and Displacements of the Uterus. In *An International System of Electro-Therapeutics*, ed. H.R. Bigelow. Philadelphia: F.A. Davis Co.

Twiss, R. (1911). Experiences of a Pioneer Electro-Therapist in Mississippi. *Journal of Advanced Therapy* 29:92.

Uwins, D. (1833). *A Treatise on Those Disorders of the Brain and Nervous System, Which are Usually Considered and Called Mental*. London: Kenshaw and Rush.

Valenstein, E. (1986). *Great and Desperate Cures: The Rise and Decline of Psychosurgery and Other Radical Treatments for Mental Illness*. New York: Basic Books.

Van De Water, M. (1940). Electric Shock, A New Treatment. *Science News Letter* 38 (20 July):42–44.

Vertinsky, P. (1990). *The Eternally Wounded Woman: Women, Doctors and Exercise in the Late Nineteenth Century*. Manchester: Manchester University Press.

Vonnegut, M. (1975). *The Eden Express*. Toronto: Bantam Books.

Wanner, A.L. (1942). Shock Therapy in Mental Disease. *The West Virginia Medical Journal* 38:107–113.

Ward, M.J. (1946). *The Snake Pit*. New York: Random House.

Warner, J.H. (1986). *The Therapeutic Perspective: Medical Practice, Knowledge, and Identity in American Medicine, 1820–1885*. Cambridge: Harvard University Press.

Warren, C.A.B. (1982). *The Court of Last Resort: Mental Illness and the Law*. Chicago: University of Chicago Press.

———. (1983). Mental Illness in the Family: A Comparison of Husbands' and Wives' Definitions. *Journal of Family Issues* 4:533–558.

———. (1986). Electroconvulsive Therapy: New Treatment of the 1980s. *Research in Law, Deviance, and Social Control* 8:41–55.

———. (1987). *Madwives: Schizophrenic Women in the 1950s*. New Brunswick, NJ: Rutgers University Press.

Warren, C.A.B., & Levy, K.L. (1991). Electroconvulsive Therapy and the Elderly. *The Journal of Aging Studies* 5:307–327.

Weck, E. (1986). Electro-Shock Therapy: Controversy Without End. *FDA Consumer* 20:9–11.

Weiner, R., & Krystal, A.D. (1994). The Present Use of Electroconvulsive Therapy. *Annual Review of Medicine* 45:273–281.

Weiner, R., Fink, M., Hammersley, D., Small, I., Moench, L., & Sackeim, H. (1990). *The Practice of Electrotherapy: Recommendations for Treatment, Training and Privileging*. Washington, D.C.: American Psychiatric Association.

Wesley, J. (1759). Preface. *Desideratum, or Electricity Made Plain and Useful by a Lover of Mankind and Common Sense*. London: Printed and Sold at the New-Chapel,

City-Road and at the Rev. Mr. Wesley's Preaching Houses in Town and Country.

———. (1790). *Desideratum: Or, Electricity Made Plain and Useful by a Lover of Mankind and Common Sense.* 3rd ed. London: Printed and Sold at the New-Chapel, City-Road and at the Rev. Mr. Wesley's Preaching Houses in Town and Country.

———. (1958). The Works. Grand Rapids, MI: Zondervan Publishing House. Whytt, R. (1765). *Observations on the Nature, Causes and Cures of Those Disorders Which Have Been Commonly Called Nervous, Hypochondriac, or Hysteric: To Which are Prefixed Some Remarks on the Sympathy of the Nerves.* London: T. Becket and P.A. DeHondt.

Wilkinson, G. (1792). An Account of the Good Effects of Electricity in a Case of Violent Spasmodic Affection. In *Medical Facts and Observations*. Vol. 3. London: for J. Johnson #72, St. Paul's Church Yard.

Winslade, W.J., Liston, E.H., Ross, J.W., & Weber K.D. (1984). Medical, Judicial and Statutory Regulation of ECT in the United States. *American Journal of Psychiatry* 141:1349–1355.

Wood, A. (1973). "The Fashionable Diseases": Women's Complaints and Their Treatment in Nineteenth-Century America. *Journal of Interdisciplinary History* 4:25–52.

Wood, H.C. (1887). *A Treatise on Therapeutics.* 6th rev. ed. Philadelphia: J.B. Lippincott.

Wortis, J. (1962). Review of Psychiatric Progress 1961: Physiological Treatments. *American Journal of Psychiatry* 118:597–601.

Wu, C.H. (1984). Electric Fish and the Discovery of Animal Electricity. *American Scientist* 72 (November–December):598–607.

Wurtzel, E. (1994). *Prozac Nation: Young and Depressed in America.* Boston: Houghton Mifflin.

Zarrow, M.R., Schwartz, C.G., Murphy, H.S., & Deasy, L.C. (1955). The Psychological Meaning of Mental Illness in the Family. *Journal of Social Issues* 11:12–24.

Zenner, P. (1883). The Value of Gynecological Treatment in Hysteria and Allied Affections. *Journal of the American Medical Association* n.v.:523–525.

Zimmer, R., & Price, T.R.P. (1991). It Ain't over Till . . . ECT, Depression, Competency, and Ethical Dilemmas. *Journal of the American Geriatrics Society* 39:438–439.

Zubin, J. (1940). Electric Shock. *Science News Letter* 40, 20 September, 380

ADDITIONAL REFERENCES FOR THE UPDATED EDITION

http://www.anxiety-depression-alternatives.com (2008)

http://www.bhs-info.com (2008)

http://www.depressiontreatmentnow.com (2008)

Gilula, Marshall F, MD and Daniel L. Kirsch, Phd, (2005) "Cranial Electrotherapy Stimulation Review: a Safer Alternative to Pharmaceuticals in the Treatment of Depression." *Journal of Neurotherapy* 9, 7-27.

http://www.hypnosecrets.com (2008)

http://www.ect.org (2008)

http://www.fullspectrumsolutions.com (2008)

http://www.electroshock.org (2000)

http://mikalina.com/Texts/amber.htm (2008)

Moore, Heidi W. (2004) "A Novel Convulsive Therapy for Depression." *NeuroPsychiatry Review* 5, Sept,.n.p.

http://www.neuronetics.com (2007)

http://www.neuronetics.com (2008)

Office of Patients' Rights, (2004).

   Electroconvulsive Therapy (ECT) Statistical Report. Sacramento, CA: California Department of Mental Health.

http://www.shgresources.com/gems/stones/amber/ (2008)

http://www.therapeutictouch.org/newsarticle/php?newsID=1 (2208)

http://www.thymatron.com (2008)

Index

About the Authors

Timothy W. Kneeland is an Associate Professor of History and Political Science at Nazareth College of Rochester. His research interests include the history of science and medicine, U.S. political history and the American Presidency. He is currently working on a history of natural disaster policy in the 1970s and revising a study of the chemist Robert Hare for publication in the *Pennsylvania Magazine of Biography and History*.

Carol A. B. Warren is an Emerita Professor of Sociology who worked at the University of Southern California for 17 years and the University of Kansas for 14. Her research interests are qualitative methods, social control, the cultural history of psychiatry, and gender. She is currently a qualitative methods consultant for a KUMC-based project on Assisted Living, and has papers forthcoming with coauthor Kristine Williams in the journals *Qualitative Sociology*, *Journal of Aging Studies*, and *Women and Health*. With another coauthor, Tracy Karner, she is working on a second edition of *Discovering Qualitative Methods* from Oxford University Press.